From Cancer to Counselor

One Woman's Journey
Through the Darkness of a
Terminal Illness

-By B. Henson-Bini

ISBN 0-7414-2184-4

Cover art: Betty (Richardson) Henson-Bini, 1984.

Published by:

INFINITY
PUBLISHING.COM

1094 New DeHaven Street, Suite 100
West Conshohocken, PA 19428-2713
Info@buybooksontheweb.com
www.buybooksontheweb.com
Toll-free (877) BUY BOOK
Local Phone (610) 941-9999
Fax (610) 941-9959

Printed in the United States of America

Printed on Recycled Paper

Published February 2005

Table of Contents

To my husband Dill and his mom Pat
for taking charge when I couldn't handle things
and to Dill, Bobbi, Patrick and Scarlett
for their love and devotion

Forward

Thank you for your interest in this book. The information you hold in your hands can change your life, whether or not you have had cancer. This book is a compilation of my personal experiences with terminal cancer, my research findings, and a collection of various other things that I hope you may benefit from. It is important to realize one truth above all else before you continue. Life has no guarantees. *Every individual is a unique creation with a specific "purpose" for living and I believe has a certain path that they must walk in order to reach their own potential.* We often become frustrated because our lives do not seem to be the way we want them. It is easy to make excuses for not taking action to change things, to blame others, and to allow fear to immobilize you; to take a wait-and-see attitude when it comes to accepting control of your own behavior and making changes that can drastically alter your life. Believe me, I know what it is like to have been a procrastinator and faultfinder. Now I like to imagine that I am the captain of a ship that represents my life. I make the decisions about how to navigate treacherous waters. I use the technology available to me, I refer to maps that have been created by people who have sailed these waters before me, and I allow the influence of my gut instincts. I have met people who gave the control of their "ships" over to another person or worse, refused to take control at all. When you do this, you are at the mercy of the sea. You are tossed about and if you reach land at all, you are probably not going to end up where you want to be. It's a better idea to plan the route towards your destination and take control of the helm.

When my oncologist told me I only had eight weeks to live, I picked my jaw up off the floor and said to myself "it's now or never" and got busy. I felt like there was something I could do to be an active participant in the fight against cancer. Let me emphasize that I was given no hope by a doctor that had already seen me accomplish things that were amazing for ordinary healthy people, nonetheless people in my "condition" going through chemotherapy, surgeries, and radiation. I went to grad school, went through a separation and divorce from a man I had spent my entire adult life with, bought a house by myself, and in the meantime got through cancer treatment alone as a single mom with two small children, very little family support and no job. After all that I graduated with honors and only missed one day of school in two years because I was in ICU waiting for my mother to die. This doctor was the same man that had praised my accomplishments, marveled at my positive attitude, and commended my fighting spirit. I knew it had to be bad for him to be so negative with me. He told me that the only hope was to radiate my whole head, which "might" extend my life slightly, with considerable risks and side effects. It wasn't much. He and his nurse both hugged me and that is how it ended. No follow up appointment. I felt like they dropped a bomb on me and then sent me home to die.

I had only been in his office 5 weeks earlier for my 90-day checkup and they said everything was fine, no cancer anywhere. They never looked inside my head, where they would have found multiple metastatic masses that had originated from the breast cancer I had been battling for the previous 2 ½ years.

This disease is mysterious. It is baffling. It is unpredictable. I do not know as I am writing this if I will live long enough to see it in print, or if I will live to be

100, but I feel absolutely positive that had I known then all the information I know now that cancer wouldn't be an issue in my life.

At present, my new medical team is astounded. Even though most of my brain at one time was overrun with cancer, I have a quality life and since I started using my own resources to fight this disease, the spread of the cancer has halted and even reversed. *They have called me "their walking miracle"*

I hope that my story will inspire you and get you excited about taking control of your own life. I want you to get busy today. Don't wait. I wish you a long, healthy, productive life and I offer you this information as what I see as my own purpose in life, to help others. Good luck to you and keep the faith!

Who Am I?

I am not a doctor, not a nutritionist, nor a scientist. I am an average person who lived an average life at one time. But that all changed when I found out I had cancer. So why is there yet another book on how to fight cancer by a non-expert? I pondered this question myself. I have no medical training and no so-called credentials to lead me through this endeavor. What I do have is compassion for others and a willingness to share what I have learned from first hand experience. If at times I seem to glide over the technical aspects of a topic, then hopefully you will understand. If you want to explore the scientific side of things in depth, then you would do well to supplement this book with one that is more scientific. My purpose is to give others like myself some hope. I like to know why things work the way they do and I make an effort to explain, but not in detail. To me, if it works, that is the most important thing. Why it works I may not understand entirely.

Because I am not a medical professional, I can't make any promises or give any guarantees. I can only tell you what works for me. I want to strongly caution you though that people with certain conditions, like diabetes and obesity need to inform their medical professionals before participating in any program that can affect the performance of the body. I know what it is like to have the doctors run out of options and to cause you to wonder what else is out there that you don't know about. Medicine is not the only option. There is a whole world out there full of remedies and hope.

If you or someone you love has this horrible disease, then don't give up hope. As long as you are breathing, there is life in you and I believe that as long as we have life we have hope. You are not a victim. The only thing that victimizes us is ignorance. *You do have some control over what happens to you.* The fact that you are reading this shows you are determined to be knowledgeable about your disease and research your options. If you read about the different types of cancer patients, you will learn that the ones who are active in their treatment are most likely to recover.

Cancer forced me to dig deep into myself and find strength and purpose I never felt before. I could no longer rely on modern medicine because even with all the technology we have today nothing could save me, according to my doctor. Because of this, I had no choice if I desired to live but to turn to alternative therapies to combine with the medicine and have hope that something I could do would work. I learned that people every day are either cured from cancer, go into spontaneous remission, or the cancer simply disappears with no explanation. I wanted to be one of those people that could share a testimony of hope with others.

It is ironic when I think about it now but on 3 separate occasions I was "given a message" about cancer. I was handed the answers long before I had the questions but I was too blind to realize the messages were for me personally. I now believe everything happens for a reason.

First, in 1985 my sister gave me a "diet" book. Its main premise was that you eat foods in the proper sequence in order to maximize nutrition. It talked a lot about vegetarianism and promoted a vegetarian diet, which I was not interested in. I read the book and was taken in by the concept, but in 1985 I felt good and looked good and wasn't the least bit concerned about what order I ate my food in. I put the book away thinking that one day it might be a good idea to give it a try.

Then, in 1999, I was standing in my bedroom ironing clothes and watching TV. I had never watched this Christian station before, but when I was flipping through the channels, I saw a physician giving a testimony about having cured herself from breast cancer. She mainly used raw fruit and vegetable juice. I was mesmerized by her story and I thought one day I would look her up again. It is amazing to me now that at that time, the cancer was probably just getting kicked up in my system then without my knowledge.

The third and final "coincidence", which I like to think of as God's final tap on my shoulder, happened with His impeccable timing. I was searching a bookstore site on the Internet and even though I thought I was in remission at the time, I found a book about fighting cancer that caught my eye. I didn't know exactly what I was ordering, but I bought it anyway and since it was a used copy, I had no idea when to expect shipment so I forgot about it. It arrived and was waiting on my porch the day I received the news that I was terminal. It was a book about nutrition. These three messages of hope are what got me started on the project of putting together a program that I could live with (no pun intended) and do on my own. It is not my intent to usurp anyone's research. I am simply sharing my story with you and the plans that I followed during my struggle to regain my health. This became my personal program of recovery.

Have you ever disregarded a gut instinct? Are you willing to consider new approaches?

Traditional Treatments

So what happens after you hear the "bad news"? Your doctor will refer you to an Oncologist (cancer specialist), or in some cases, a surgeon to take the cancer out if possible before treatment.

Here is what happened to me. First I had a palpative exam manually. The mass was looked at by the sonographer on an ultrasound. Then I had a mammogram. The doctors were suspicious and did some preliminary tests. They examined my blood and attempted a needle aspiration. This is a type of biopsy that can be performed very simply and quickly and usually can give results right away. In my case, however, they had difficulty performing the test and the results were inconclusive. Because of the lack of results from all the tests I had, they went ahead and did a lumpectomy, or surgical biopsy. In some cases they just take a tissue sample but in my case they removed the entire mass and sent it to pathology. I had what is referred to as neo-adjunctive therapy. That is where you start chemotherapy before surgery. Then they took the lymph nodes out from under my arm. I had chemo again, followed by radiation. The oncologist put me on hormonal therapy daily. I then had my gallbladder removed and later had a complete hysterectomy. I was operated on by a neurosurgeon who cut into my brain and removed a tumor. I had radiation again followed by chemotherapy. In between all those procedures I went through physical therapy twice. In summary, I had 5 surgeries in 3 years, 3 rounds of chemotherapy, 8 months of weekly blood tests, radiation twice, hormonal therapy for a year, physical therapy twice, and I lost all of my hair three times! I have had a dozen or so scanning procedures including heart, bone, and CT scans, MRIs, and x-rays.

For your information, there is a glossary at the end of this book that defines many terms with which you may be unfamiliar. I always took notes when I went to the doctor so

I could go home and read them and then if I wasn't clear about something, I could call his office and clarify it or wait until my next appointment. I also kept notes at home about odd twinges and things that would happen to me so I could take the questions with me the next time I went.

I would like to express something here that I feel very strongly about. *Do not think of your doctor as infallible.* He or she is human. Always remember that. My surgeon told my dad many years ago that he did the repair work but only God could heal. I trusted my surgeon to the extent that I did everything he said. But when it came to treating the cancer, first I asked my oncologist what he would do if he was treating his wife, then I made the decision about what I wanted to do based on my own research. If you ever become dissatisfied with medical staff, remember this; they work for you. You pay their salaries. Furthermore, I have expectations of dedication and compassion from my medical team and I have not hesitated to ask questions, complain about service, and even switch professionals because of dissatisfaction.

I remember one day going in for chemotherapy and the nurse that was to start my IV had a bug bite on her ankle that she kept scratching until it started bleeding. I insisted on getting up immediately and talking to the head nurse about it and after that, I never saw that woman there again. There are some things you just do not have to put up with.

My mother was the opposite and swallowed every pill, accepted every treatment, agreed to every surgery or procedure, and took all her doctors' advice, even when she felt in her "gut" otherwise. I have been given prescriptions before and thrown them in the trash afterwards because of research I would do when I got home with them. My doctor originally gave me anti-seizure medication to begin taking before I flew over the Atlantic. The reasoning was that if something happened to me midair, nothing could be done until I reached mainland. I refused to take the medication because it was the type of drug that you would have to take continuously once you started and I didn't feel like I needed it. I won't take pain pills because they are hard on your liver.

My doctor recently tried to give me anti-inflammatory drugs for the symptoms I have due to long term steroid use that resemble rheumatoid arthritis. I told him I would rather suffer through the pain because he said it would only last a few months. I will not take a drug unless I know exactly what it does in my body. I would advise the same for everyone. I have taken chemotherapy and am aware of the devastating effects it can have on your body and so I don't want to add to the damage with other drugs. Additionally, I have worked as an addictions counselor and I know how highly addictive some of the narcotics are (mainly tranquilizers, sleeping pills, and pain pills) which doctors are freer to prescribe to the cancer patient. My theory about this is that some have a lack of concern about addiction because they don't expect their patients to live very long.

Please don't get me wrong, I love my doctors and are grateful to all of them for their efforts with me. If it were not for a couple of doctors who really believed I was "worth saving", I probably wouldn't be alive now. I had to search for a medical team that I liked and trusted. I would never rely on just one doctor's opinion. There is always something that can be done. New cancer treatments are being discovered all the time. I believe that traditional cancer treatments do work on the symptoms. And I believe that they can buy us time while we try and develop plans to help our bodies heal themselves from the underlying cause of the disease. But keep in mind a couple of things.

Even though we call surgery, chemo, and radiation "traditional" medicine, the original medicine was no chemicals at all, only natural products and faith…and the pharmaceutical business is a $7,000,000,000.00 (yes…that's 7 BILLION) per year business. You can patent a drug and sell it but you cannot patent a natural substance. There is not a lot of money to be made in natural substances as compared to drugs. Interesting, huh?

What types of treatments have you received? Were they effective? Do you have to go through treatment again? Are you willing to augment your traditional therapy with alternatives?

The ugly "C" word

Cancer. Just hearing the word makes people shake their heads in pity and think of death. I used to be one of those people too. When I found out my doctor suspected I had breast cancer, I went to my sister-in-law for support. I'll always remember what she said to me. "The word cancer doesn't frighten me now". She had previously had a mastectomy and was undergoing reconstruction.

Let's see… I had two uncles die from cancer, two aunts die from it and both my parents had experienced it, along with many relatives and people that I knew, yet I can't ever remember thinking I might get it. I was one of those invincible people that thought nothing serious would ever happen to me. Disabilities and disease only happened to others. Boy, was I wrong. Not only was I wrong about myself, but the first time I walked into the "chemo" room at the cancer treatment center, I was in for a startling realization.

There were multiple rows of stations, each with a recliner, blanket, television, magazines, and an IV rack, and most of them were occupied. Some patients were bald, some young, and some old, of varying nationalities. Wow. I didn't realize how prevalent it was especially in my home community which I considered to be modest in size. I was in for an education all right.

I remember one time asking my doctor, "What do you think cancer is?" to which he gave me the technicalities of cells mutating and multiplying, etc. I said, "no, I know what it does, I just want to know what you think it is." He shrugged his shoulders, shook his head and said that no one really knew what it was. He is a doctor and not a scientist. He only knows what the medical community teaches. I started my research that day.

I learned that one in 7 women in the U.S. will get breast cancer in their lifetime. One in 2.5 Americans will develop cancer of some form. The younger you are when you are diagnosed, the worse your prognosis is. Cancer is one of our nation's leading killers, second only to heart disease. The U.S. has a higher incidence of cancer than any other country.

If you look in the Encyclopedia Britannica, this is what you will find under the topic of cancer: "cancer is a group of more than 100 distinct diseases characterized by the uncontrolled growth of abnormal cells in the body." According to the Merriam-Webster dictionary, it is defined as "a malignant tumor of potentially unlimited growth that expands locally by invasion and systemically by metastasis." Okay. But what causes it?

Write down what you think causes cancer.

The suspected causes

First let's consider the body's metabolism and what happens when you eat. When you take a bite, the food begins breaking down as you chew with your teeth and salivate in your mouth. When you swallow, the chewed food makes it's way down to the stomach where the stomach acids immediately start breaking it down further. The gallbladder and liver secrete bile in order to further digest the food. As it begins its way through the intestines, the nutrients are picked up by cells in the blood stream and then the blood passes through the liver to filter out the unwanted waste products. Then the filtered blood continues its job in the body contributing to the creation of new cells.

We lose 10 million cells in our bodies every day. Most of them die, some are defective or diseased, and some are cancer cells. That's right. Cancer cells. But because our liver is the superhero of our immune system, it can usually filter out all the unwanted stuff in our bodies and what it doesn't get, the white blood cells come out in force and attack the intruding material. That's how it's supposed to work. In with the good, out with the bad.

Now there are multitudes of theories of what exactly causes cancer and just as many products on the market designed as cures or treatments. When I examined all of those that I came across in my research, I established my own conclusion. *It all boils down to this: when your body is exposed to too many toxins or poisons either from it's own metabolism or from the environment and it cannot process them adequately, the waste is recycled in the body and used in forming new cells.* Your body is therefore making new cells out of defective material and thus you have a final product that is also defective- a less than perfect cell.

A few thousand of these probably wouldn't cause you any great detriment. But think about this. A million human cells can rest comfortably on the top of a pinhead!

My original lump or mass in my breast was about the size of my pinkie fingernail, according to the surgeon who removed it. Every day our bodies fight these infections and foreign bodies by destroying them with white blood cells. But just like my checking account, when you spend more money than you have, you are running a deficit. It is the same with our bodies. When you tax your immune system over its limit, it can't handle all the work and so some things just don't get done. My belief is that cancer (any type) is caused by the body being overloaded with poisons.

When I was a little girl my dad was a plumber and would let me go to work with him sometimes. I remember him talking about how deadly sewer gas was and so that is why he would stuff old cloths in the hole in the floor when he removed a toilet. Just think about that for a minute. Where does sewer gas come from? Human waste. Waste products that were formed when your body stripped all the nutrients from the food that you have eaten. It makes perfect sense that waste inside your body must be eliminated because it is toxic or poisonous.

Look around you at your environment. Do you know what is in the water you are drinking? Bathing in? Have you ever gotten behind a vehicle at a stop light that was pouring exhaust into the air you were breathing? Do you always carefully wash your produce when you get home from the grocery store? Remember spending summers at Grandma's house that was painted with lead paint? Did the authorities have to renovate your school when you were a child because it found asbestos in the ceiling? What about the "bug truck" that would go slowly through the neighborhoods in the summertime and spray this awful smelling stuff to kill the mosquitoes- did you have one of those like I did? There are pollutants all around us. Our planet is filthy. Even something that seems so pure like rain falling from the sky can kill our most beautiful trees. Sounds pretty dismal, huh?

Now ask yourself. What did you eat today? Write it down in the space below.

Now think of all the pollutants you may have been exposed to today. Write them down in the space below.

Toxic Blood

Let's talk about all the carcinogens in meat products- mainly hormones to make the animal grow faster to be ready for slaughter sooner than is natural, hormones to make animals produce more milk than they naturally do, so dairy farmers can make more money off each individual cow, and hormones to egg laying animals to increase the production of the eggs from what the animal would naturally hatch. Notice the reference here to the unnatural nature (see the oxymoron there?) of all this. I was particularly interested in hormones because the breast cancer that I had was ER- Estrogen Receptive and was caused by too much estrogen in my body. Before doctors stopped recommending Hormone Replacement Therapy I already had suspected that it might contribute to developing breast cancer. When the risks were publicized I felt certain of my conviction. I know you've heard about how it's not wise to disturb the balance of nature and this is a perfect example of how what seems harmless can become huge when you tamper with it.

These hormones gather in our bodies, especially in our fatty tissues and our intestines. Because meat has no fiber, we get constipated and that rotted food just sits there. Because our bodies are designed to circulate nutrients for building new cells, our blood picks up acids and other toxins from this spoiled food and distributes them throughout our bodies. Think about that image the next time you order a steak. We won't even begin to discuss the cruelty involved in raising meat animals to satisfy those American cravings. I have tried in the past to research that topic, but when I see those pictures of animals locked up in such tight quarters they have deformities it makes me sick.

In addition to the fact that meat is unhealthy because of all the toxins it contains, when the digestive system acts on it, it turns to acid. Some theories about the causes of cancer attribute the unbalanced ph level in the body to the formation of disease. Because our bodies are mostly alkaline, eating foods which turn to acid in the body can throw this balance off. What foods turn to acid in our bodies? Mostly proteins, like meat, eggs, and dairy products.

All these toxins are supposed to be removed from the blood by the liver. It acts as a filter to clean your blood. Imagine your air conditioner or dryer filter to be clogged with dust and dirt to the point that the air will not circulate adequately, and the air that gets by is not being filtered at all. Many times I have smelled stale air and checked my air conditioning filter and it is clogged, or I've gone out in the backyard and noticed lint that had escaped from my dryer vent because of a clogged filter. It is the same with our livers. Not only do our livers filter poisons out of our blood, but the liver is the main organ involved in our immune system. *Do you want your immune system so beaten down by poisons to render it unable to defend you from disease?* Me neither.

So how do you get the protein your body needs? I remember one time when I was student teaching that I allowed a girl who was failing U.S. History to do a current events paper for extra credit. She chose vegetarianism. About midway through her paper a particularly rude young man interrupted with arguing that you had to eat meat in order to get protein. He showed the class his muscles and they whistled and applauded. I allowed this chaos to play itself out until the room finally settled down and in that moment a divine revelation hit me. I looked out over the class and asked, "Where does a racehorse get protein?" Not a sound in the room. "Seeds and grasses," I said. Case closed. I gave the girl an "A" on her paper. In my mind, it was extraordinary because she presented the class with a topic that caused everyone to think. Any time you can cause people to be more open minded I think you have done something great. Hopefully this book will cause you to question your old beliefs.

Disease isn't random. There is always a cause. Some diseases are acute (they happen suddenly) and some are chronic (they take a long time to manifest and can last a lifetime). Most people find out they have terminal cancer very suddenly and some even die immediately in my opinion from the fear that they are going to. But cancer is not an acute disease. It can take years and years for it to accumulate in your body enough that it forms a mass or tumor. The regeneration of healthy tissue is time consuming but so is the formation of unhealthy tissue. Cancer is a systemic disease. By this I mean that it is created by the failure of a system, mainly our immune system. Our focus should be on the entire system that is affected.

Dirty intestines and a dirty liver contribute to the dirty blood that makes us sick. Before we can focus on getting well, we have to do some serious housecleaning inside our bodies. It doesn't matter if you are so inspired by this that you start eating right today because by now your intestines are probably so dirty that they can't function properly. Normally, your intestines absorb substances like vitamins and minerals from things that you digest (I call them "things" because not everything in you is food- think about drugs for example). These nutrients are what is made available to the rest of the body for making new cells. That is where the importance of eating high fiber foods comes in. It is a good idea to supplement your diet with natural fiber to keep the foods you eat moving through your intestines and cleaning them out along the way. But if your intestines are so clogged that they aren't working right, then what is being used to form new cells? It is vitally important that we cleanse our bodies and provide it with proper elements to create new cells. Our body's God given ability to create new healthy cells is what heals us, causes us to grow and allows us to produce babies from single eggs. *The creation of new unhealthy cells causes us a lot of problems, but the one we need to worry about the most is cancer.*

You might present the argument here that you know someone who has always lived a healthy lifestyle before getting cancer, or that children with cancer cannot possibly have destroyed their bodies in such a short time. Please answer this question. Where did you get your genes? I got mine from my parents when their bodies were making new cells and replenishing the old ones in their reproductive systems before I was born. All my DNA was given to me by my parents and their bodies. What if they had clogged filters? Then I would have been "made" from their unhealthy, mutated reproductive cells. I think about that when I see the checklist on the medical evaluations that ask you to check off diseases present in your family. *Family. Genes. Cells. Nutrition. It's all related.*

Write down your feelings about eating meat for protein.

Acidosis

When the liver filters the blood it removes toxins that are acidic and it produces enzymes, which are alkaline. Acidity and alkalinity are opposites. The balance of the two is referred to as your body's ph balance. When your body's ph balance is too acidic, it is in a state called acidosis, which occurs more readily in people with diseases and is often fatal.

The kidneys extract the acid to help keep our blood in an alkaline state. If you have ever known anyone who has had kidney stones, that is what happens when your kidneys try to process an over-abundance of acid in the urine. Acid is also present in the toxic wastes in our intestines. The colon will redistribute these acidic poisons back into the body if it is not cleaned out regularly. The lymphatic fluid picks up the wastes that are dumped back into the bloodstream and carries it throughout the body. When the fluid is acidic, it is more difficult for it to move freely and so the chances of these poisons being stored in the lymph nodes is higher in a state of acidity. *The condition of metabolic acidosis occurs when the body is in a constant state of acidity and can lead to death.*

The body tries to balance itself by pulling alkaline minerals from the blood. If there are none available, the acids will accumulate in the cells. All this knowledge should lead you to be concerned enough about your body's ph level that you want to be sure it is in an alkaline state. If all this isn't enough, then consider that research has indicated that cancer cells grow in acid. That is enough to make me want to be sure that I give my body the best chance of being more alkaline than acidic. You can test your ph balance by simply using ph paper found in the pharmacy. If your ph balance is off and your body is acidic, you can drink sodium bicarbonate to reduce the acid in your digestive tract and then supplement your diet with extra calcium to counter it at the cellular level. Taking calcium prevents the body from pulling calcium out of the bones to help balance the acid.

You can also choose foods to eat that are lower in acidity. These are most fruits, green vegetables, peas, beans, lentils, spices, seeds and nuts. Acid forming foods include meat, fish, poultry, eggs, grains, dairy products, and legumes. Ideally, your diet should be 40% acid forming foods and 60% alkaline.

Write down the foods that you usually eat that are acid forming foods.

Metallic poisoning

Metallic toxins interfere with the absorption and transport of nutrients. *The presence of these metals can be deadly if there is a high enough concentration.* Low concentrations make you sick. Think of lead poisoning and how many children it kills every year. I can remember two instances of coming in direct contact with harmful metals. The first was when I was a child and dropped a glass thermometer. The glass broke and the mercury inside balled up and went rolling across the kitchen floor. I thought it was neat so I picked it up with my bare hands and stared at it. The other contact that I had that I remember is when I bought a historic home. The kitchen walls were wooden boards that were painted bright yellow and the paint was peeling off in places. I tried scraping it off but it was too tiresome so I bought a heat gun and melted the paint away. I used a dust mask at first but it didn't fit right and kept slipping so I finally took it off. I was inhaling the fumes of lead paint without realizing it. I was pregnant at the time. When it hit me what I had done, I got a sick feeling in my stomach. It was too late to do anything about it I thought.

Back then I had not heard about Chelation Therapy. This is when a doctor injects a chemical into the bloodstream that can cleanse away excess metals (minerals). The substance adheres to the metallic molecules and then they are taken out of the body in the urine. Deadly metals that you may come in contact with include lead, mercury, arsenic, and cadmium. Nowadays you can get herbal tablets that work in the same way as Chelation therapy. They are available in pharmacies, health food stores, and online.

Think of the metallic poisons you may have been exposed to.

Parasites

I was appalled to learn that humans have intestinal parasites or worms. I remember having to take a stool sample to school in the fourth grade so it could be checked for worms but I think that was the last time I thought about it until I started doing research on cancer. There are a variety of parasites that can invade the body such as tapeworms and roundworms just to name a couple. I have read testimonies from people who have expelled 24-inch tapeworms! People around me that I told this story to held up their hands and said, "No more! I don't want to know!" Although I could appreciate their humor, I didn't feel that way. If there was a living organism inside me I wanted it gone. I can just imagine a scene from a sci-fi movie where a horrid creature tears through my abdomen while I am screaming, "Get it out!" They take up residence inside your body when you eat food that contains invisible eggs, or from touching something contaminated and putting your hands near your mouth. The smaller varieties can even enter through the pores in your skin. A "Vermafuge" is something that you ingest to rid your body of parasites. These are usually herbal combinations that you can purchase online or in health food stores.

How would you feel if there were parasites in your body?

Candida

When I first started my regimen, I began developing white blotches in my mouth. My doctor informed me that I had "thrush" caused by an over-abundance of yeast in my system. He prescribed a fast-acting medication for me that I didn't want to take because of the strain it puts on the liver but because I was getting ready to travel internationally, I had to take care of it right away. After investigating what the cause of this was, I learned that it was called Candida Albicans and is caused by a proliferation of yeast in the body. I had always suffered from yeast infections (once a month as a matter of fact) so it didn't really surprise me. *Candida is a product of the fermentation of glucose or sugar in the body and provides and environment in which cancer cells thrive*. But how do you get rid of it? Diet is the main culprit (of course). Sugars and high fructose foods like fruits, and breads with yeast can feed the yeast and cause it to grow.

In my case, the thing that tipped the balance was the high doses of supplements that were in a base of yeast. Also, I suspect that the Selenium supplement I was taking had a role because it is a type of yeast. When I came back from my trip I again developed these sores. I had learned from the Internet that Tea Tree Oil or Melaluca Oil can be used to combat thrush. It is a topical herbal infusion that is not supposed to be taken internally but I did it anyway. I would dab the spots in my mouth with a cotton swab dipped in the oil (it tastes like turpentine) and then would drink a small glass of water, ingesting what was in my mouth. Doing that in combination with cutting back on my yeast containing supplements caused the thrush to disappear. Months later Candida returned in the form of a vaginal yeast infection. I decided this time to try an herbal product specifically designed to attack Candida and it worked. I would recommend using a combination of the herbs and diet.

Have you ever had a yeast infection? Thrush? If yes, what did you have to do to get rid of it?

Dehydration

Our bodies are made up of mostly water. Our breath contains a lot of water. Go outside on a cold day and watch your watery breath turn to steam every time you exhale. Imagine how many times you exhale in a day! Every cell we have depends on water to keep it regulated. Our body systems need water too. Your mouth needs water for its saliva production. Your eyes need water for tears. Your brain is bathed in cerebral fluid. Your nasal passages are moist so that substances you inhale will stick to them and not go into your body. Your intestines need water to help them stay supple and pliable. Your liver and other spongy organs are porous and contain a lot of water. You can live for a long time without food but your body can only survive for about three days without water.

Every secretion in the body is carried by water. Bile, spinal fluid, and blood plasma (just to give you an idea) all contain mostly water. Have you ever tried to give blood or have it tested and the nurse is having a hard time finding a vein? Or have they found a vein but the blood is not flowing freely? Ask them about this. They will tell you to drink more water.

Have you ever felt bloated like you were retaining water? Maybe your body is afraid to lose the water it has because you are in the habit of not giving it enough. Water regulation is like food regulation. When you diet and try to lose weight, your body recognizes that you are cutting down on your calories and in the beginning it slows down its metabolic functions until it is sure you are not starving it. This is a defense mechanism to fight famine. It is the same with water. The less you consume, the harder your body tries to keep its reserves in case of a drought. The more water you drink, the less water your cells retain.

Water is needed to transport oxygen and other nutrients throughout the body. *You have to have water to excrete the toxins from your body.* Your urine, sweat, mucous, and fecal matter are mainly water. If your fecal matter is not wet, then it is not the consistency it needs to be. Humans need to drink at least eight glasses of water a day. Humans with cancer need to drink more! The best thing to do is to go out and buy either a water purifier that is hooked into your sink, or to buy a pitcher with a filter. I have the inexpensive pitcher that I keep in the refrigerator so the water stays cold all the time and I don't have to worry about using ice made from tap water.

Do you drink enough water? How many glasses (8 oz) of water do you drink per day?

America the cancer-ful

When I was in Greece on my honeymoon I was in culture shock. I have always had a healthy appetite. As a child I would embarrass my family when we went out to eat at one of those all-you-can-eat places. Back then, if you wanted more, it wasn't as simple as going to the buffet because there was none. You had to tell the waitress what you wanted and they would cook it to order. People would tell me that I wouldn't always be able to do that because it was bad for me. But I did it anyway. When it came to food I admit I was somewhat gluttonous. I grew up in the South, where fried foods were normal for every meal and we used lard and pork fat in just about everything we cooked. We cooked our vegetables "to death" and hardly ever ate anything raw.

My first morning in Greece, I waited for my hostess to make a suggestion for breakfast. She didn't. We made coffee and drank that instead. Then I waited for her to make a suggestion for lunch. She didn't. By then I thought I was going to pass out. She was a model at one time and never ate that much, but I found myself nibbling on the kid's donuts by about 1 pm. At dinnertime, she said she was ordering a feast. I thought to myself, "Thank God." We walked a little ways from her home into a small restaurant and ordered take out. Except for the meatballs that she ordered for the kids, it was mostly vegetarian. But it was very satisfying to me.

(By the way, the Greeks don't raise their food animals the way we do. I heard a story when I was there that they actually take goats by boat to tiny islands and let them eat fresh grass and reproduce over the winter without human contact. Then in the spring, the herders retrieve their increased population of healthy goats, and make dairy products out of their milk, which is untreated by chemicals).

As our honeymoon progressed and we saw more of the country and became conditioned to their customs, I had learned a few things. First, we didn't eat anything I don't think while we were there that didn't contain olive oil. Either it was cooked in it, drizzled on it, or stirred in it. As far as fat goes, the only fatty foods we were exposed to were grilled meats, dairy products (especially yogurt and goat or feta cheese), and desserts. There were some common American fast food places but even at those the menu was different than the ones in the U.S. You didn't drink sodas or tea unless it was hot tea. You would drink water, fruit juice or coffee and of course wine. You could walk into any café and order an orange juice and get a giant glass of freshly squeezed juice at about half the price of a cup of coffee!

I finally confessed to my friend that I was hungry in the morning and she showed me how to make tzaziki, a sauce or dip made from primarily cucumbers and yogurt. Every morning I began by having bread dipped in tzaziki. Even the bread had little fat. It was dried, like crackers and if you wanted it soft, you would sprinkle water on it. My friend's husband would eat this with chopped tomatoes and goat cheese as a snack. I wasn't thrilled about eating dairy products, but being so far away from home did make eating well difficult. Before we went to Greece I told my friend what I was doing and she told me not to worry, that she had a juicer. When I got there however, it was more like a blender and I did try it but couldn't stand the texture of the finished product and so unless I drank fresh citrus juice, I didn't consume any while there.

When we did eat in Greece, it would be mostly salads and vegetables and the vegetables would either be raw or grilled. Plus, there are not as many conveniences as in the US. The grocery stores are tiny places and if you want fresh fruits and vegetables, you have to go to a market. There are very few pre-packaged foods. No soup or canned vegetables in the grocery stores. There is not a fast food restaurant on every corner. It is no wonder to me that Greece has one of the healthiest populations in the world.

When I came back to the U.S., I started researching other cultures. I examined European, Asian, and North

American cultures and just as I suspected, the Asian countries were the healthiest, followed by the European (Mediterranean countries were healthier than inland countries) and the North American continent was the unhealthiest, not only because the U.S. is in it, but because we have so influenced our neighbors that they eat like we do. *Anytime a country begins to "Americanize" with fast food restaurants and typical American food, its population becomes less healthy.*

Do you ever eat ethnic food? How does eating food originating from another country satisfy you? What is your favorite? Why?

Alternatives

Many alternative therapies focus on nutrition. Did you know that medical doctors are not required to have extensive knowledge about nutrition? Most medical universities offer one mandatory course in nutrition and that's it. I remember when I first heard I was terminal; I was desperate to get my hands on a plan that I could start immediately. I wanted to go to a holistic center where I could learn better nutrition and alternative treatments. My insurance wouldn't pay for it and in order for them to reserve me a spot, I was required to put up a deposit of $24,000.00. That's twenty-four thousand dollars for a deposit! I wasn't going to allow myself to be victimized by a society that only seems to care about people with money. I decided the only alternative therapy I could afford was to design a program for myself from the research I could find. I will go through my reasoning for this plan below but here it is.

I used a very common sense approach that was a combination of all my research. This was a 3-point plan:

1) *Cleanse the body*
2) *Feed it nutrients*
3) *Love myself*

I was stricter with myself in the beginning because I was afraid it would not work if I wasn't but I don't do all of these now. I've relaxed a little. I seldom do enemas and I do eat "normal" cooked food, mostly vegetables. I make sure that my diet is mostly live foods with a high water content. I still juice almost every day but usually only once or twice a day. I feel like some of the changes are lifelong, like healthy eating, exercise, supplementation, and nurturing myself. Here is an example of a typical day for me when I was trying to cleanse the toxins out of my body and it is what I would suggest:

Enemas 1 coffee enema in the am, 1 plain water enema in the pm

Juicing Fruit juice in the morning and Vegetable juice in the afternoons (as much as you can drink up to 8 glasses a day) for at least two weeks without solid food, longer if possible. (When you begin eating meals, continue to drink juice whenever you desire. I usually make juice now for breakfast, have it as an afternoon snack, or both).

Supplements a multi-vitamin with minerals, beta-carotene, selenium, calcium, vitamins C, E, B complex, A (water soluble), acidophilus, zinc, and fish oil

Water purified or filtered, drink it all day long

Chlorophyll in powdered form that you mix with liquid, once a day

Psyllium (a laxative powder made of natural fiber), once a day

Herbs ginger, ginseng, garlic, tea tree oil, herbal hot tea (a couple of times a day), an anti-inflammatory combination, parasite cleansers, Candida cleansers, Chelation combinations.

Exercise

Relaxation

Prayer and Meditation

Visualization

Positive Affirmations

Working towards my goals

Psychotherapy intermittent throughout the entire time

Journaling

I started every morning by giving myself a coffee enema. Only when I felt like my bowels were cleansed did I feel like I could continue with my day. I would then drink a cup of herbal tea. I heat my water first, then put in the tea so it's medicinal properties are not destroyed. I may drink green tea, ginger tea, red clover, rose hips, or a variety of herbal combinations that are available at my health food store. I would then make my fruit juice and take about half of my supplements (I would be too full to take them all). Around midday I would drink my oxygen drink made with the chlorophyll powder and vegetable juice. Throughout the day I would carry around my thermal "jug" of cold water. I would make juice as often as I could and would drink that all day long. I always listened to music to lift my spirits or provide a mood setter for whatever activities I was doing. I would walk my dog around the neighborhood. Sometimes I could only go to the end of the street pushing a wheelchair because I was so weak and unbalanced that I wanted it with me in case I needed it to get back home or just sit down and rest. When I came home, I would drink my fiber drink (psyllium) and take some more supplements. In the afternoon I would make vegetable juice and drink that. If I was particularly hungry I would eat a carrot, apple, banana, or sliced tomato (bananas helped ease my cramps).

Eventually I started eating salads and then sprout sandwiches. All day long whenever it occurred to me I would think to myself how I was doing good things and was helping my body heal itself. I repeated these positive affirmations to myself all the time. Every day I would decide upon one thing I would accomplish. It might only be doing 10 stitches in a crocheted scarf I was making. But I would set goals however small they might be and I would make sure I accomplished them. I would give myself an enema at the end of the day. If I could take a bath, I would run water to fill the tub while I gave myself a dose of tea tree oil. Then I would light candles all around, play soft music, use an herbal bubble bath or Epsom salts, and just relax. When I lay down at night, I would meditate, pray, and visualize my cancer being destroyed as I drifted off to sleep.

When you have a full day of doing everything you can to destroy the cancer cells and heal your body it is very rewarding.

Write down your feelings at this point about the program.

Cleansing the body

Enemas

Sounded pretty gross to me too when I first started getting advice from every direction that this was the thing to do to get started cleansing my body. You know, some people pay hundreds of dollars for professional colon cleansings but I would much rather do it for just a couple of dollars in the privacy of my own home. What I do is spread a towel on my bed to lie upon (in case of an accident) and begin by relaxing. It's a good idea to warm the liquid you are using slightly to bring it at least to room temperature before you use it. I always run the container under hot water in my bathroom to do this. You can use disposable enemas or buy an enema bag. I will lie down on my left side. If you have ever seen a picture of your colon, this will make sense to you because of its shape. If you point the tip towards your belly button you will have the right angle for insertion. Just go slowly. Squeeze the liquid gently. When you have done this, wait as long as you before expelling your bowels. At first this really hard for me to do but eventually you will be able to hold the liquid in.

I buy my enemas from a pharmacy and wash the containers thoroughly in hot soapy water to refill them for the coffee enema the next morning. You can buy enema bags but I found it convenient to just buy the disposable ones. The bags hold a lot more and really provide a better cleansing but I really didn't think I could hold that much in long enough to empty the entire contents of the bag. At first I would do a couple of enemas every day. Now I do them about once a week or so. Oh, by the way, using enemas frequently will rob your intestines of good bacteria and you need that so it is a good idea to take acidophilus when you are using enemas because it helps replace what you lose.

Why coffee? In my research I discovered that coffee enemas have been used for a very long time medically to cleanse the colon and help detoxify the body. Evidently, the stimulants in the coffee encourage bile production and help the liver rid itself of toxins. My husband always has a pot of coffee brewing and so I would just let this cool down and use it the next morning. Brewed coffee is the only kind that will work by the way. The ratio that I used was 3 parts distilled water to one part brewed coffee.

Don't be surprised at what comes out of your body. Remember, it may be material that has been in your system for a long time. In the beginning, my bowels expelled a black material for the first few times. My lungs also began expelling toxins in mucous. This lasted for about four days. At first, I thought I had pneumonia. I coughed constantly and was coughing up chunks of phlegm and blowing mucous out of my nose all the time. When it went away, I realized that it was probably nicotine build-up from when I had been a smoker. Then one day I was minding my business doing other things and without warning, I felt something being expelled from my body through my rectum. I hurried to the bathroom to find my intestines had shed a huge amount of mucous. It was probably between a half-cup and a cup of this material and it was a ball of slime about as big as my fist! I know that is more information than you wanted but I didn't want you to be "creeped out" as my daughter would say if this happened to you.

I realized when I started this that I had suffered from being chronically constipated all my life without even realizing it. Cleaning out my intestines, using fiber, and juicing helped me get on a regular schedule where my body was expelling wastes the way it was supposed to. Before, I might have one bowel movement every three days or so. After I started my program, I would pass soft fecal matter very easily about three times a day!

Write down your reaction to using enemas.

Exfoliation

Your body secretes wastes or toxins in the following ways: through the rectum and urethra in feces and urine, through the skin via your pores and sweat glands in perspiration, and through the nose and mouth in aspiration and mucous discharge, and through the eyes in tears. I never thought of exfoliation of my skin to be of any importance other than beauty. Imagine in a day's time what substances you may come in contact with and not even think about. Toner in the copy machine, dirty doorknobs, bacteria in restrooms, on shopping carts, on elevator buttons, on mail, etc. All these have the potential to cling to your skin, be absorbed by your body and add to the toxins already present there. I am aware that this is extreme but I believe that every little bit helps.

I know that even though there supposedly has been a study done on antiperspirants and their susceptive link to breast cancer that came out inconclusive; I personally don't use antiperspirants but deodorants instead. It just makes sense to me that if my body wants to excrete poisons through my sweat and I am using a chemical under my arms that keeps me from sweating, then those poisons are either blocked in my lymph nodes, stored in my breast tissue, or continue on circulating my body to try again, passing my brain on the way. It may not have any effect at all, but I choose not to take the risk. I remember when I went through eight months of chemotherapy and stopped, that my body had a funny odor. Nothing I could do would get rid of it. Looking back now, I realize that it was trying to get rid of the poisons from chemo and the cancer cells that it killed through my pores.

That brings me to exfoliation of the body. By simply using a loofah instead of a washcloth in the shower or tub and showering often and immediately after you exercise, you are sloughing off dead cells and debris and you can eliminate outside pollutants and help inside ones have an easier escape route out of your body. If you don't know what a loofah is, it is a natural scrubber for your skin that you can buy very cheaply in most pharmacies and even in those cheap discount stores.

Do you own a loofah? Do you use it?

Exercise

I had a hard time deciding where to put exercise in this book. If you want to be good to yourself, exercise is a great stress-reliever. Most people however do not exercise to relieve stress. They force themselves to exercise to lose weight or become physically fit.

One of the biggest ways you can prevent heart disease is to exercise. Our concern in this book though is cancer and so I decided to put it under cleansing because that is what it does for us to help us fight cancer. Exercise helps us sweat. Sweating is one of your body's ways of secreting waste materials. When your body temperature is raised high enough, fat cells begin to burn. Fat cells are storage sites for excess calories and happen to be one of the favorite places that our immune systems like to dump toxins, away from vital organs. *By burning these fat cells, we are eliminating stored toxins from our bodies*. There is no point in my going into the other benefits of exercise because there are thousands upon thousands of books about it.

I strongly suggest that you place exercise at the top of your list in your plan of attack. I had weight gain from steroids creep up on me so fast that it felt like one day I was skinny and the next I was fat. Changing my dietary habits made me feel better and I am sure helped in my weight loss after stopping the steroids, but exercise might have made it progress faster. By the time I go to the point that I wanted to exercise, I was so bloated and heavy that my knees made it nearly impossible to stand and do anything and lying down was extremely uncomfortable for me because of problems with my equilibrium. I went to physical therapy to try and recover some of my physical strength but no matter what they did, I suffered from soreness that was so bad that I could not walk for days afterwards and was in constant pain. I had to give up physical therapy because even that was too much for my weakened body.

I had to start out by doing exercises on my own while sitting in my chair and then eventually I started doing rotations on my exercise bike. Let me try and help you understand the condition that I was in. At first I didn't have the strength to get on the bike, period. Then when I managed to pull myself up to sit on the bike, my sense of balance was so messed up that I felt like I was going to fall off the side. I had a lot of edema (swelling) in my head, combined with the damage from having cancer in the portion of my brain that controls motor skills. My first attempt at riding the exercise bike my goal was to do one rotation. Just one. Eventually I built up to about 5 minutes and then I started walking. Because I didn't walk very steady, I would push my wheelchair around the neighborhood with the dog leash strapped to it!

The medical university I was a patient at was conducting a study on the effects of exercise on cancer related fatigue and I decided to participate. I was in the walking group and had to walk at least 30 minutes, three times a week. At first I could only do 10 but it didn't take long until I was able to do 30. My dog became my exercise buddy and I cannot tell you how I looked forward to being able to exercise by walking in the fresh air after so many months of not being able to leave the house. If you want to test your mettle against depression, try sitting inside for months on end with no sunshine on your face! Especially when you love the outdoors and are accustomed to being outside a lot.

If you have the ability to walk or participate in some kind of regular exercise then by all means do. You never know when you may lose that ability. Not only does it provide us with multitudes of health benefits, but also for the cancer patient it does something we need very badly. It gives us a reason to look forward to getting out of bed in the morning.

How much exercise do you get in a week?

- ❑ Going to the mailbox and grocery store is your exercise. You always take the elevator because when you walk up the stairs you get winded. You only sweat when you are hot. Exercise? What's that?

- ❑ You walk the dog down the street when it's not raining. You mow the lawn and trim the hedges. You wash the car in the driveway when it needs it. Exercise? Hahahahaha, yeah I remember that. It was the stuff they used to make us do in P.E.

- ❑ You play with your kids outside, walk to the corner store, park away from the mall, and take the stairs when you can. You consider yourself an active person but you just can't find time to exercise.

- ❑ You make an effort to do Tai Bo at least once a week, bowl in a league, and you go for a brisk walk sometimes after dinner. You think you do okay but you realize you could do more on a regular basis.

- ❑ You walk/jog every other day and on rainy days you ride your stationary bike for at least thirty minutes. You have as many exercise clothes as you do normal everyday clothes. You are proud of your accomplishments.

- ❑ You work out at the gym, run 5 miles on the beach every day after stretching, and take a spinning class. When you go to the beach you want to swim, surf or play volleyball. You consider yourself an athlete.

Nutrition

Most people would agree to a link between cancer and diet or nutrition. It makes good sense to me that we Americans are so sick because of our poor diets. Other nations do not have the fatty diets that we have and their populations are healthier. The American diet is referred to as the SAD. This stands for the standard American diet but it is ironic that it is indeed very sad. It is loaded down with fat and too much protein from meat, eggs, and dairy products. Other countries have diets lower in fat and eat much less than we do. Especially when it comes to meat. Have you ever been to an authentic Chinese buffet? Notice all the beautiful variety of vegetables cooked with a little meat as a flavoring. The vegetables are quickly sautéed and appear nearly the same as they did when they were in their natural growing state. Now think about the typical American buffet. It usually has a meat station- roast beef, ham, sausages, steak, fried and roasted chicken and it is likely the most popular place in the restaurant. You will probably also find tons of casseroles, vegetables that are usually canned and covered with butter and salt, lots of breads, and salad bars loaded with things like potato salad and coleslaw and of course a variety of fattening dressings. And don't forget the huge dessert tables which we do not even need to discuss. When you drink a beverage, how often is it herbal tea or water? Do you ever have fresh fruit juice or do you drink a lot of coffee, sodas and iced tea?

Okay I'm not going to beat this point to death. I think we already know that too much fat and protein isn't good for us. A large majority of people have tried high protein, low carbohydrate diets to lose weight. Does it work? It works for a lot of people. Is it healthy? Let me ask you this. If you eat eggs and bacon for breakfast and drink a glass of milk, have a little salad with cheese, covered with your favorite dressing and chicken for lunch, and eat a steak and green beans cooked with ham, washed down with diet soda for dinner, do you think it is healthy? Yeah, I know. Restaurants are changing their menus to include low-carb items. It is because they are in business. They have big marketing departments that are always looking for trends. They are jumping on the bandwagon of a public fad, in hopes of making money. They are executives, not nutritionists. I've known people who have eaten like this for long stretches of time and it greatly concerns me. I try not to talk to them much about it, because they get mad at me when I do. I think it is okay to cut down on carbohydrates in the form of bread, cereals and grains, but I don't believe compensating by eating more meat is a good thing.

I was in the grocery store recently and heard someone asking the deli worker if they had low carbohydrate wraps. The whole nation it seems is on a high protein, low carb diet. The worker made a comment to me that she didn't understand that diet craze, that people should know that eating that much meat can be dangerous. I said that when more people began dying from heart attacks the government would eventually figure out that it was linked to this program and start putting out warnings. Please use your own logic when choosing foods to eat. It is so obvious to me that this diet is unhealthy but it just goes to show you how Americans are more concerned with the way they look than anything else.

Now for some people, this diet is recommended for a short period of time, because it does seem to cause weight loss and can be especially beneficial for obese patients with health issues that need to lose weight quickly for medical reasons. *But in the long term eating too much meat is very dangerous.* This throws your body into Ketosis, which I learned in high school biology, is a condition that can cause death. Just like our bodies, these meat animals have livers and immune systems that take all the toxins they can and process them. What they can't filter out is stored in the fat cells in a concentrated form and when you eat that meat you are eating unknown chemicals that animal has ingested in its lifetime. Not only has the animal's liver been trying to do its natural duty, but also it has been given a huge amount of hormones and other additives to the animal's food. It can't possibly filter out all that so it stores it for later but later never comes.

Let me tell you some facts about animals for food (please keep in mind that I would rather eat a big, juicy slab of rare beef than anything else in the world). First of all, proteins form acid and ferment in the human body, mainly because when you eat a big juicy steak your body doesn't know what to with it so it tries and tries to digest it, unsuccessfully and it rots inside your body. Why doesn't your body handle meat well? In my opinion, we weren't designed to be meat-eaters. As much as I hate to admit it, I think it is the truth. Look at all the meat-eaters of the world like tigers, alligators, and eagles. They are predators. Their bodies are built for speed and power. They have claws or talons to take the prey and to help pull the meat apart, and/or sharp teeth or beaks like knives for tearing tough meat and they also have amazing jaw strength. Plus, they have keen eyesight to help them as they hunt and catch their prey. They eat their catch raw, bowels first because that's where all the nutrients are. Where did these nutrients come from? That's right, plants that their prey had already eaten and digested conveniently for its killer.

Have you ever known anyone with TMJ problems? TMJ stands for temporomandibular joint, or the jaw joint. The jaw pops out of joint when you eat. There are almost 11 million sufferers of this in the United States alone. I have known someone who had this and had to have her jaw reset and wired and could no longer eat meat because she didn't have the jaw strength to chew it. Our jaws do not seem to be built to withstand a lifetime of chewing meat.

Besides all of this, even though I like my meat rare, eat sushi, and eat raw oysters, the idea of eating raw flesh, intestines, organs, and drinking warm blood is disgusting to me. I would not go through all that in order to eat one meal. I would simply pick berries with my berry-picking fingers and

I would eat leaves with my grinding teeth and I would eat fruit that entices me with its scent when it is ripe and colorful. The smell of food attracts us, just like bees to flowers. It is supposed to do that.

When have you ever smelled an elephant and thought that smell was appetizing? When food is in it's natural state, the only foods that lure us are the fragrant ones that grow out of the earth, not the furry, leathery or feathery ones. I bet you are thinking that you like the smell of meat while it is cooking. Me too. It makes our mouths water. Think about the smell of sizzling steak. It is almost addictive to us. What would you rather eat, a grilled meat, or a raw vegetable? Of course a grilled meat because of the smell (unless you are a vegetarian and if you are kudos to you). And once we get a whiff of that aroma of cooked meat, it is very easy to over eat also. So why would we rather eat a grilled meat than a raw vegetable? Because cooked meat smells stronger. When our olfactory glands sense a strong food odor, it triggers a biological response in us that makes us desire to eat. We automatically choose foods that are the highest in calories because our appetites are programmed that way.

Remember, we are advanced beings with the ability to reason and hardly resemble our early ancestors, but our natural instincts still rule us in certain areas. We have a strong will to survive, we are constantly experiencing the "fight or flight" syndrome in our daily lives, we have a sexual drive that enables us to propagate our species, and our bodies' metabolism is regulated by the same systems that the first humans had. In our modern day lives making a profit is the key element in the production, shipment, and merchandising of food. Meat companies "dumb us down" by tempting us with the way the meat looks after it has been cooked and it garnished and plated nicely. In the "old days" we had to butcher our meats. The butcher's case would be stocked with whole dead animals, like they still are in Greece.

I went with my friend and her 2 yr. old son to the market one day in Greece and when we approached the meat counter, the little boy shrieked, made an ugly face, and covered his eyes. Skinned, bloody rabbits were lying in a row for sale, next to the whole plucked chickens. It really was frightening. One night when we went out for dinner, while we were eating our food, a truck drove up, parked beside our outdoor table, and two men unloaded a dead lamb to take into the restaurant. Believe me, those two incidences stuck in my head for a long time and it was a while before I wanted to eat anything other than fruits and vegetables.

Nowadays, our produce is shipped before it is naturally ready to eat. Fruits and vegetables picked before they were ripe do not have much of a smell. Grocery store tomatoes and cantaloupe are textbook examples. But have you ever eaten a homegrown, just-picked ripe tomato, still warm from the sun? In my opinion, they are heavenly. What about the sweet, juicy, colorful cantaloupes? Same thing. Their flesh is aromatic and tender, not like those hard grocery store ones. I love going to the farmer's markets. The aromas are tantalizing. I always buy more than I need of fresh fruits and vegetables. I just can't help it. We always follow our noses and eat what is most pleasing to us- that is our natural tendency. Raw meat does not smell very good. If we smell foods in their raw natural states we are attracted only to fruits, vegetables, greenery, berries, and flowers. I believe that the closer we mimic the way nature intended us to eat the healthier we will be.

I have included some vegetarian recipes at the end of the book for you so that you will be able to enjoy that same feeling of anticipation and temptation without all the protein and toxins from meat. They are some of my favorite recipes.

The food we consume today is mostly convenience food. If it isn't fast food laden with grease and far too many calories than our bodies need for energy, then it is what you think is a healthier choice food sprayed with chemicals to keep it preserved. You can cook at home of course but keep in mind that your fruits and vegetables are grown in pesticide and insecticide contaminated water, your meat animals are given growth hormones to make them mature faster and lay eggs quicker and produce more milk. Even if the natural foods that grow from the earth are not poisoned with chemicals, they do not contain the nutrients they should because the soil has been turned and reused so many times that it has no nutritional qualities left.

My advice when purchasing produce is to find hydroponic (grown in water) varieties and organic ones (certified that they are grown without the use of chemicals). This is especially important with raw foods that you normally eat the skin of. If you can't find them, then I would wash the others thoroughly with mild soap and water and if you cannot remove the waxy coating, I would peel them.

How many times per week do you eat out? What do you typically eat?

Juicing

The Food and Drug administration has published what it considers the minimal consumption of fruits and vegetables in our diets. So how can we possibly get the nutrition that we need on a daily basis? It is nearly impossible to eat all those, and besides the FDA only suggests minimal standards. The cancer patient needs more. One way to get enough vitamins and minerals is in a concentrated form- juices of the foods and not the bulk of the foods themselves. I am not talking about the stuff on the beverage aisle in the grocery store. I am talking about buying fruits and vegetables and extracting their juices. Bottled or canned juices have been pasteurized and that process robs them of their life-giving enzymes.

Once you have tasted fresh squeezed juices, it is very difficult to drink anything else. There is something very pure and natural about juicing that just feels good. It gives you energy when you are weak and quenches a deep thirst that nothing else can. It can fill you up to the point where you don't even want all those bad foods, which can assist you in losing weight too. My kids love fresh juice and that makes me very happy.

Juicing is the best way to start this program not only because of the nutritional value of fresh juice, but because of it's detoxifying effects on the body. The first two weeks of the program I would fast from food and drink juice instead. The juice is easy for the body to digest and helps the liver out by allowing it to focus on cleansing the blood and assisting the immune system rather than being tied up with digestion duties. When you are allowing your liver to take a break from digestion and concentrate solely on immune functions, the likelihood is higher that it will turn its attention to destroying your cancer. I wanted to be sure that my liver was free to work on the cancer cells in my body and so I juiced every day for about a month, occasionally eating live foods towards the end. Be sure that when you are juicing, you are also using enemas. A lot of poisons are in your system when you start and are produced from your body "throwing out the garbage" when you start giving it healthy alternatives. These toxins need to be flushed out so they don't get recycled in the body.

I would buy a professional juicer that allows you to insert whole products so that you do not have to stand there and pre-cut your fruits and vegetables. I had one of those machines with a small chute and my back got so bad that I couldn't stand there and cut things up. For awhile I would take anything that needed preparation to the kitchen table and cut it up sitting down, but I didn't always feel like doing that and on those days I wouldn't have any juice at all unless someone else made it for me. Also, you want to be sure and drink your juice almost immediately after making it because part of the point is to ingest live enzymes and they have a very short life once you juice them. I would always drink my juice within twenty minutes after preparing it.

Have you ever had fresh juice? Do you have a juicer?

My favorite juice recipes:

Garlic

1 carrot
2 tomatoes
1 stalk celery
2 radishes
1 clove garlic

The garlic in this one also has intense properties to help cleanse the blood and eliminate Candida fungus from the body. Cancer thrives in a fungal environment.

Green juice

1 cucumber
2 stalks celery
½ clove garlic
1 T. powdered chlorophyll drink mix

This one provides chlorophyll to the body and oxygenates the blood to be carried to all the forming cells. Cancer cannot survive in an oxygen-rich environment.

Pineapple/Orange

Fresh ¼ pineapple
2 oranges
1 slice of lemon
1 apple

The enzymes in pineapple help the pancreas and take a load off the liver in digesting. This allows the liver to free up other enzymes to seek and destroy cancer cells in the body and provide nutrients to newly developing cells so that they mature into healthy cells.

Carrot/Celery

4 carrots
3 stalks celery

This is the beta-carotene booster. It seeks out free radicals in the body that turn normal cells into cancer cells. Research also shows it can inhibit the development of newly growing cancer cells.

Watercress Beet

4 tomatoes
2 carrots
1 whole beet
3 watercress leaves

Beets add a bright color and texture to the juice and are a liver purifier. Watercress provides calcium and chlorophyll.

Cucumber

2 whole cucumbers
1 stalk celery
1 slice onion

This is good with chlorophyll powder also.

Apple carrot juice (this is my 9 yr. old daughter's favorite)

2 apples (I like one sweet apple and one sour)
One small piece of ginger, maybe ¼ inch in diameter
4 carrots

Has digestive enzymes that aid the liver in digestion and also has beta-carotene

V-7 (my 10 year old son asks for this almost every day)

2 large carrots
½ peeled cucumber
1 stalk celery
½ clove garlic
1 red tomato
¼ green pepper
½ c Alfalfa sprouts

This tastes similar to the commercial vegetable juice and contains powerful antioxidants, beta carotene, and chlorophyll

If you are interested in specific juice combinations that target specific areas of the body, then you can research what ingredients you need on the Internet and in the libraries. My juicer came with a recipe booklet, which was very helpful. My kids love to experiment by using a variety of fruits and vegetables. Beets are a lovely color, as are carrots. Green apples and celery are too. Watermelon and cantaloupe make scrumptious juice. Things like grapes and strawberries can add flavor to your fruit juice by using just a few. Peppers and garlic add zest to vegetable juices. Have fun with this. If you only drink one kind all the time, eventually you will become bored with it. In the beginning, I would only drink carrot juice. I drank so much carrot juice that I turned orange! Literally, my lips and hands especially, but also my skin had an orange tint to it. Like they say, you are what you eat!

Live Foods

Any food that is raw is considered a live food. Our bodies use enzymes only found in live foods for creating life in us. Our bodies can reproduce cells without enzymes, but they are not fully functioning. Each cell has a specific job to do and needs enzymes to give it the maximum potential to be a specialized cell that can perform a specific duty. Cancer cells are not specialized. The only thing they "know" how to do is divide. And they are very good at that and do so at an alarming rate because that is their only function. They don't have regulatory mechanisms that tell them when to stop. By giving our bodies more enzymes, we are improving the chances that our new cells will be able to be specialized cells and have all the necessary components to perform at top efficiency.

The liver usually provides digestive enzymes but for those of us with cancer, the liver is too busy trying to deal with the enormous amount of cleaning it has to do. If we ingest these enzymes then we can provide additional assistance to our livers and digestive functions so that they don't work so hard. This feeds our bodies these essential enzymes without having to depend solely on the liver to produce them. *Live foods also give us vitamins, minerals, fiber, and water.* Examples of live foods are salads and fruit medleys. The more raw food you eat, the healthier you are. Raw food also contains fiber that helps cleanse the colon of unwanted waste residue. Fruits and vegetables in their raw state are the best sources of nutrients that we have.

I would get really hungry when I first started juicing because of the appetite stimulants I was taking and so I would occasionally eat whole live foods. Later after I felt like my body was cleansed (when I stopped expelling "yucky" stuff from my bowels and my bowel movements became regular and effortless) I slowly added meals but I would make sure they were at least 70% water containing foods like vegetables. Since our bodies are made up of mostly water, it is important to keep that water intake up or we get dehydrated. New healthy cells can't be formed by a body that is dehydrated so keep your water intake up not only with liquid that you drink but with live foods which contain natural waters full of nutrients.

Eat freely from this list of raw foods after your 2-week juice fast:

Apples
Alfalfa sprouts
Asparagus
Avocados
Bananas
Beets
Blueberries
Broccoli
Cantaloupes
Carrots
Cauliflowers
Celery
Cucumbers
Garlic
Grapes
Grapefruit
Honeydew melons
Kiwis
Kumquats
Lemons
Lettuce
Limes
Mangoes
Nectarines
Onions
Oranges
Peaches
Peas

Pears
Peppers
Pineapple
Plums
Radishes
Spinach
Squash
Starfruits
Strawberries
Tangelos
Tangerines
Tomatoes
Watermelons
Zucchini

Name ten foods from this list that you would eat.

Try making a vegetable salad and squeezing a lemon on top, drizzle a little olive oil, and herbs such as minced garlic, oregano, basil or dill. After you have been juice fasting, it will be healthy and filling. When you get hungry, munch on sliced apples, oranges, plums, tomatoes, cucumbers, radishes, broccoli, cauliflower, carrots, or celery. Just pick a fruit or vegetable that you like. All these will add bulk and fiber to help clean out your intestines and they won't contain all the toxins of foods such as meat, eggs, and dairy products. Only add a scant amount of these high protein acid-forming products to your diet if you wish after you have been on the program for a while and are satisfied with your results of toxic cleansing (at least a month). It sounds hard I know but it is well worth the results. I was fascinated the day that a skin cancer on my arm just dropped off. I had noticed it started getting dry and flaky before but when it actually fell off dead, I knew I was doing something right!

If you keep a bag of prepared salad and veggies in the fridge and some fruits in a bowl then they are readily available and easy to access. You want to be able to grab them when you are really hungry and stay away from other foods at first. Can't stand the thought of eating cold fruit for breakfast? Try sticking a half grapefruit under the broiler for a few minutes, or baking some apples with a little cinnamon. Warm peaches, pears, and plums are good too.

Steamed or slightly cooked foods to add a few days after you start eating solid food again:

Artichokes
Broccoli
Brussel sprouts
Cabbage
Cauliflower
Celery
Collard greens
Eggplant
Green beans

Kale
Lima beans
Mushrooms
Okra
Onions
Pea pods
Prunes
Rutabagas
Squash
Sweet Potatoes
Turnips
Zucchini

After you have juice fasted and begun re-introducing solid raw food to your system, for breakfast you can begin to have grain toast or waffles, oatmeal with raisins or apples, multi-grain English muffins or bagels without feeling guilty. For breakfast, try whole grain cereal or oatmeal with soymilk and bananas. Have a salad or a multi-grain veggie sandwich for lunch and a dinner, which is made up of at least 70% water containing foods like fruits and vegetables. Try to eat only grilled lean meats or fish and small portions of those. Drink fresh juice in between meals and drink lots of water throughout the day. I would try to consume mainly juice and live foods the majority of the time.

My usual grocery list now:

Apples
Oranges
Carrots
Celery
Tomatoes
Cucumbers
Lettuce
Greens
Olives
Garlic

Ginger
Sprouts
Other fresh fruits and vegetables
Raisins and other dried fruits
Canned tomatoes
Canned vegetables
Salsa
Applesauce
Brown rice
Dry beans
Whole grain breads
Whole grain cereals and pasta
Frozen vegetables
Lean meats like chicken breasts and pork chops
Canned broth
Olive oil
Honey
Herbs and spices
Tea bags

I have small children who love foods like pizza, hot dogs, hamburgers, etc. When I began introducing more salads and vegetables, much to my surprise, there was no resistance. I started substituting things like salmon and grilled chicken breasts for hot dogs and burgers and surprisingly they started telling me how much they loved the good food I was cooking for them. When your kid comes up to you in front of people and asks for broiled fish and spinach for dinner, it is a day to celebrate.

Write down a list of foods that you can buy from the grocery store.

Herbs

When I visited my friend in Greece, I passed a lot of time sitting on the balcony overlooking the sea and reading. Because she is an esthetician (skin care specialist) she had a lot of books about herbs and skincare. I was amazed at the properties that herbs have. We talked a lot about the similarities between having healthy skin on the outside and what it takes to be healthy on the inside. I was fascinated by some of the new things I learned. Below I will give you a list of herbs and how they are beneficial to the cancer patient, according to my research.

Please keep in mind that some herbs can be very dangerous. For example, did you know that the heart medication called Digitalis is actually a flowering plant? Consult an herbalist or someone who has knowledge of herbs before you try them naturally. Of course some companies make it very easy by packaging the products in the safe amounts for you. You can find teas and topical skin ointments usually in grocery stores or pharmacies and also the packaged form of the herb itself, in a bottle that resembles vitamins. Check with your doctor too because some herbs are as strong as pharmaceutical drugs and can interfere with your medications.

This section can be extremely overwhelming, or at least I was overwhelmed with all the options and not knowing what to do. I only include this as a topic of interest to get you started on you own research.

Aloe Vera—the juice promotes bile flow and is very alkaline, the gel promotes skin health

Alfalfa—pulls toxins out of cells, alkalizes the body

Apple—liver stimulant

Astragulus—increases white blood cells and can help the immune system

Barberry—fights Candida

Basil—oil is a natural insect repellent

Bitter candytuft—digestive tract

Black Walnut—fights Candida

Chamomile—anti-inflammatory

Clove—fights Candida

Co Enzyme Q10—removes toxins

Dandelions—promote bile flow

Echinacea—immune and lymph stimulant

Elderberries—promote sweating, laxative

Feverfew—encourages more blood flow to the brain

Figwort—lymphatic swelling

Flax—eases constipation and liver congestion

Garlic—an antioxidant, also strongly fights Candida, acts as a Chelation agent

Gentian—liver stimulant and fights Candida

Ginko Biloba—increases blood supply to the brain and protects against free radicals

Ginseng—immune system stimulant

Goldenseal—bile stimulant

Lavender—promotes bile flow and helps ease pains in the brain and head

Licorice—detoxifier

Milk Thistle—liver cell renewal and fights Candida

Mint—promotes sweating

Oatmeal—lowers cholesterol, fights depression

Olive leaf—fights Candida

Onion—can use on insect bites

Pau D'Arco—fights Candida

Peony flower—anti-spasmodic

Plantain seeds (or psyllium)—sluggish bowels

Primrose—promotes sweating and is a calming agent, kills cancer cells

Pumpkin seed—fights Candida

Raspberry—cleansing laxative

Red clover—lymphatic swelling

Rhizome (also called Mexican wild yam)—bile stimulant

Rhubarb—laxative

Rosehips—vitamin C

Sage—memory loss, promotes bile flow

Strawberry—liver tonic

Tea tree oil—fights fungus and bacteria, cold sores

Thyme—fights Candida

Willow bark—anti-inflammatory

Wormwood—fights Candida

Verbena—liver restorative

Viola—anti-tumor, lymph swelling

Yarrow—promotes sweating

Green Ginger Tea

The kids would rather drink this than soft drinks!

Fresh ginger root
2 T. Honey
2 lemons
8 bags Green Tea (can buy this in the grocery stores in bags just like the black tea)

Fill kettle with distilled water. Peel a ½ in. chunk of fresh ginger and drop in kettle. Heat water to almost boiling and then steep tea bags for 10-15 minutes. Pour into pitcher with honey and squeeze in lemons, adding fruit to pitcher. (You can make this hot or cold).

Green tea is a powerful antioxidant that can prevent new cancer growth and ginger is a natural liver detoxifier and digestive stimulant. Also, the hot bitter bite of ginger helped me eliminate toxic mucus from my lungs during my detoxification and helped me breathe and sleep easier.

Again, here is another section that I had trouble deciding where to place. It fits in all three categories. Some herbs cleanse the body. Some herbs are highly nutritious, and some just smell so good that we can use them in our personal care. You can find herbal recipes for almost every kind of cosmetic product. Right now herbal products are very popular and you can find them in any pharmacy or discount store. For better nutrition, herbal teas are wonderful as are the fresh herbs themselves, sprinkled on foods. Herbal supplements can be used to help the body properly eliminate toxins and support liver and immune function. Shampoos, deodorants, bubble bath, hand lotions, soaps, astringents and toners are just some of the few things that you can buy made with herbs. Whenever you have a choice between using a natural, herbal product and using a synthetic, man made one, I would always choose the herbal one. Here are some terms that you might find helpful in knowing their meanings when you are trying to make sense out of the herbal jungle.

An infused oil is an oil mixed with herbs. To make your own, you can combine in a jar your herbs and oil and leave to sit for at least 24 hours. Sunflower oil is a good oil to use for this.

An infusion is different. It is a tea that you make with herbs and boiling water.

A tincture is medicinal and used topically as an antiseptic and it is made with natural alcohol and water and herbs. Mix ¾ alcohol with ¼ water.

A cream is a thick lotion that can be made with glycerin, water, and herbs, heated gently for 3 hrs, strained, and stored in jars.

Ointments are made from petroleum jelly melted in a double boiler, mixed with herbs and strained.

A steam inhalant can be made by adding herbs to boiling water. If you do this, you can tent your head with a towel to keep the steam in but be careful because it is hot so you don't want to get too close.

Natural soaps can be made from herbs at home and make great gifts. This is done by using soap flakes, or glycerin. I would stay away from lye because it may be toxic.

What herbal products do you use now? What can you replace with herbal products?

Supplements

What is an antioxidant? Antioxidants are substances that attack cancer-causing particles in our bodies called "free radicals". Free radicals are electrically charged molecules that seek out other molecules to bind with. When they attack your healthy cells, they cause damage that can lead to all kinds of diseases, including cancer. This process is called oxidative stress. Free radicals are formed by our body's natural metabolism and they are also present in the atmosphere.

It is highly important that you take antioxidants to help your body defend itself against the attack of the free radicals. Even though fruits and vegetables contain antioxidants, we don't typically eat enough to insure that we are getting the amounts we need. Most of your supplements will contain antioxidants but each has its own specialized effect on cancer.

Again, just as with herbs, don't let this section bog you down. If you take a multivitamin, it makes things easier and then you can pick and chose what you want to add. Many of us take vitamin supplements already. If you do, I think that is good because you will already be in a routine of doing this daily. I will go through the list of vitamins that I use but you will want to get a copy of a vitamin book and do some research on your own to decide what is best for your condition. This is a list of the supplements I take and why I take them for anti-cancer purposes. Please note that many of these provide a lot more benefits than I describe here.

Vitamin A- a fat-soluble vitamin that helps cells reproduce normally so that they can continue their specialization. I take water-soluble vitamin A because at high levels it can be toxic and the water soluble is more easily metabolized by the body.

Vitamin B-There are several B vitamins and usually they are sold collectively as a supplement. I take a B complex which contains all the B vitamins. Vitamin B1 is also know as Thiamine and is needed to help the body break down its nutrients (fats, carbohydrates and proteins). Vitamin B2 is Riboflavin and is needed by the body to help process protein and fat. It also can provide antioxidant properties. B8 is also called folic acid. It assists the body in forming DNA molecules. It is needed by the immune system to help in the production of red blood cells.

Vitamin C-This vitamin is the most popular defense in the cancer community. For years, people have sought out vitamin C therapy to assist them with fighting cancer. Although most medical doctors in the U.S. will scoff at this idea and therefore not provide vitamin C therapy, there are places you can go that will give you injections of it in concentrated form. When I was first told I was terminal, I called my doctor's office and asked the head nurse where I could get injections of high doses of Vitamin C. She told me that she didn't know of any place but it didn't matter because it wouldn't help me anyway! It scares me to think of what she may be telling other patients less knowledgeable about nutrition. Little does she know that Vitamin C is a powerful antioxidant and inhibits the spread of cancer. I started taking oral supplements in high doses instead. I would take 10,000 milligrams of it per day!

Vitamin D-Typically, this vitamin is combined with calcium. This is because of its function of regulating the amount of calcium in the bloodstream. It also helps form red blood cells and can help cells differentiate, which reduces the cancer risk

Vitamin E- a powerful anti-oxidant and can help repair tissue that has been damaged by radiation.

Fish oil- omega 3 fatty acid, which is an anti-inflammatory and also increases blood flow to the brain. It may also help reduce the risk of metastases.

Copper- an essential mineral that assists in hemoglobin production and various enzyme reactions.

Selenium- an essential trace mineral for normal functioning of the immune system and thyroid gland. Incidences of cancer are lower among people with higher selenium blood levels.

Zinc- trace element that helps baldness, DNA synthesis growth and wound healing and proper function of T Cells (the white blood cells that destroy cancer).

Co Enzyme CQ10- enzyme that may reduce the risk of breast cancer and help the cells in their metabolism.

Calcium- we think we get enough calcium when we drink milk and eat dairy products. I didn't realize before I started my research that calcium is more available to us and more easily absorbed by our bodies in plant form. Live foods provide loads of calcium and do not turn acidic in our bodies like dairy products do. When we drink milk or eat dairy products, the calcium in them is only made available to us after our bodies try to counteract the acid by pulling calcium from places like our bones. To prevent this, it is much easier to eat calcium-containing live foods and to supplement with calcium tablets. Non-dairy foods which contain calcium include beans, greens like bok choy, spinach, turnips, kale, collards, and mustard greens, oranges, canned fish with bones like sardines and salmon, fortified cereals, soy milk, tofu, almonds and oysters.

Chlorophyll- our cells have to have oxygen in order to live. Cancer cells die in the presence of oxygen and it is important to do everything we can in order to make sure our bodies are getting enough. It is vital that you learn how to breathe deeply. Also, exercise helps in this area because oxygen is distributed to our cells when we are burning those calories. In brain cancer, chemo drugs have a hard time reaching the brain because of the blood brain barrier. This is like a "safety-net" membrane around the brain that is designed to discourage toxins from entering. The amount of blood reaching the brain is limited because of this. I felt like it was important for me that whatever blood was reaching my brain to contain a lot of oxygen. I began taking Chlorophyll to raise the oxygen level of my blood. I also ate a lot of greens and especially alfalfa sprouts because they provide a high percentage of oxygen when you eat them.

Name the supplements you currently take and list the ones you do not have.

Loving yourself

Do you like who you are? I realized years ago when I started going to therapy that I didn't like myself very much. If I would have had a life threatening disease then, I probably would not have tried to fight it because I really didn't feel like I was worthy of living. My therapist picked up on this right away. She told me to remember what it was like to be a helpless little girl and just imagine that this child still lived inside me with all her fears and insecurities. She told me to wrap my arms around my body as though I were hugging myself. She suggested that I do this every day and promise my inner child that I would love and protect her. The first time I did this, it was very emotional. I realized that I had abandoned her a long time ago and she had been afraid all these years because she was alone. When I was told I had cancer, I promised her that I would do everything in my power to fight this disease and keep her from dying. That was an act of love towards myself. This concept may sound strange to you but it is highly effective.

I believe that in everything we do we should search for ways to make ourselves happy and do things out of love for ourselves. This would include feeding our bodies healthy diets, not taking drugs or alcohol, giving up smoking, exercising, and pampering ourselves often. I am not talking about spending a lot of money going shopping, etc., I am talking about the freebies that we can do at home. It is amazing how you can begin to feel more worthwhile just because you devote a little more attention to yourself for a change.

How do you feel about going to therapy? Have you ever seen a therapist?

Exercise

Exercise is a way to be good to your body. Most women equate exercise with drudgery and don't look forward to it at all. This is a great way to de-stress. Especially if it is yoga combined with soft music and candlelight and followed by a nice hot bubble bath! If you are home bound as I was for several months, even getting out of the house and taking a spin around the yard in your wheelchair can lift away the blues! I talked about exercise in the section on detoxification but exercise can lift your spirits too. *When you exercise, your body produces endorphins which are chemicals that cause you to feel pleasure*. If you want to find an alternative way of relieving pain, try exercise.

Think of an activity that you would like to do to relieve stress.

Religion

At the risk of offending some readers, I have chosen to talk a little about my faith. My reason? I could not have taken on this challenge alone. There were very long stretches of time where not a single person would visit me. I had times that I felt very desperate with no one to talk to. By talking to God, I learned to trust Him more. Throughout my treatment, I found myself on a spiritual journey that would lead me back to the faith that I had as a child. I realized when I started adhering to a stricter regimen how little self-control I had.

I would let the least little thing send me into a panic. I had to learn when I had children to do the "count backwards slowly from ten" technique to stop me from losing my temper with them. The year after I was first diagnosed with cancer I was mostly alone and had a lot of time to self-reflect. I had never learned how to forgive others and I read a lot of literature about forgiveness and how harboring resentments not only causes you mental and emotional pain, but can affect your physical state as well. I had to "teach" myself how to forgive others. I did a lot of growing personally during that time and I strengthened my relationship with God so much that it became so indwelled in me that I was constantly aware of Him working in my life, arranging various things in His amazing ways.

We get so busy in our modern American fast-paced lives that we miss a lot of spiritual moments that we could be experiencing. It is easy too as a cancer patient that once you finish your treatments and are told you are in remission to want to take a break from all that thinking and just live. I know what it is like to be constantly burdened with thoughts and responsibilities all the time. My experience was that once I knew that there had been cancer in my body, there was always a hint of a lingering fear in the back of my mind that it would come back. If you stay focused on the positive and your healthy relationship with your Creator and your purpose in living, it is easier to be aware of the little ways that our lives are directed and the paths we would best be served by walking. I know that I felt broken at times in my life and I had to tell myself that God was in control. I imagine a potter who is dissatisfied with his vessel, smashing it to pieces and using the broken shards to reconstruct something new, adding more water and squeezing really hard. Occasionally after kneading the ball of clay it has to be slammed on the hard table to soften it up and purge the bubbles out. Can you imagine the pain that clay must feel? If God is the potter and I am the clay, I must go through this pain in order for Him to create a work of art in me. This image allows me to feel like my life will be better than ever at the end of this experience (live or die) and that there is a very good reason why I am going through these trials. I am given these images when I am still and quiet and contemplative. I try to always keep one ear available for that tiny little voice that directs me and I would advise you to do the same.

Churches or places of worship can be one of the best support systems in your life. Let's put aside for a moment the reason we are there- our beliefs. I can remember being intimidated by churches until I worked in one. The people there are human just like us and they want to serve others. Sure, there are scandals and such, but again if you focus on the positive, you can overlook those things. It is like anything else. You get out of it what you put into it. *Do you see how this is a constant theme in our lives?* It always works that way.

I was bummed because when the kids' dad and I divorced, I joined a church near my new home. I didn't have much of a chance to make any new friends because either I was so tired all the time, that I only went to Sunday worship services and nothing else, or I was sick and couldn't go at all. I watched the people from my mother's church constantly doing what they could to help and support her. They cooked food and took it to her, showered her with small gifts, constantly prayed for her, wrote to her, called her, brought her flowers left over from the worship service and the Sunday school lessons that she missed, and during her surgeries would come to the hospital and wait with the family. Those people really knew how to have a good time in their worship services. It was a highly charismatic church and was mainly unstructured in the way they approached worship. There was always a message, but if the spirit moved and people were being touched by God, the service could last all day. I used to love going there because you weren't restricted to stay in your seat. You could cut loose if you felt like it, dance, sing, shout, clap, and raise your hands toward the heavens. I always had a wonderful time when I attended that church but the one thing that kept me from enjoying to the point that I wanted to become a member was the intolerance there for other beliefs.

I began reaching out to my church and communicating with them. They began praying for me in their prayer meetings. I began receiving cards from other members. I started receiving phone calls from the pastor to check on how I was doing. The associate minister brought communion to my house for me. We were invited to a Thanksgiving dinner they had in the fellowship hall and if it were not for that, we wouldn't have celebrated Thanksgiving at all because the kids were away with their dad and I certainly didn't feel like cooking Thanksgiving dinner. At Christmas they took up a collection and gave my husband and I a generous amount of money to help us with presents for the kids. When I was finally able to begin going back to church, I had already established a relationship so that I didn't feel like a stranger. I felt like it was my church family and I was grateful for the help they had given me and the hand of love and friendship that they had extended.

I am a Christian but I do not believe that one branch of Christianity is better than any other. I admire other religions as well for their teachings about peace and harmony. Like I said before, I am from the south and we are in the "Bible Belt". I have been to many churches in my life and I have experienced many different kinds of faith. I have seen people treated like they are demon possessed for reading books about other beliefs. It is one thing to me to share the goodness of your faith with someone who needs it, but yet another to have an attitude of elitism and try to force others to believe that your way is the only way. This is humiliating and inflicts further pain, which can cause people to close themselves off emotionally for protection. I think it does more harm than good.

In my opinion, the truth cannot possibly revealed in our lives on Earth because that is what faith is all about- believing in that which you cannot see. There is not a single person alive that fully understands how God works. There is not a single person alive that can tell you for certain that there is a God. You have to be convicted of the belief yourself. I believe this can only come after a spiritual awakening, or by studying Christian principles until you are satisfied they are meaningful to you and you want to adopt them because you see the truth in them. I don't believe you simply say a prayer and you are changed into a different being. It is highly individualized to me. I believe in grace and mercy but I also believe that your actions in life speak volumes as to your devotion to God. A lot of people don't agree with me and that is okay. I understand. But don't condemn another for their beliefs because you are not in a position of spiritual authority. I am a spiritual being and my spirit can only be judged by God. I think some people are not aware that they are passing judgment on one another. I believe that religion is a choice and that always searching for truth as an open minded individual is a sign of intelligence.

However, personally I believe in Christ and I choose to be a Christian. I believe we should all search for the style of worship that brings us closest to God. I became Catholic as an adult because I was so moved by the beauty of the rituals. I loved the icons, the rosary, the holy water, the candles, the incense...I could go on and on about the things I loved about the Catholic church. But in the Catholic church you can only receive holy communion or the Eucharist when you are not in a sinful state. Because they do not condone divorce, you can never remarry unless your spouse dies. If you remarry you are considered to be committing adultery and therefore cannot partake of the Eucharist. To me this is unfair and appalling. I no longer was accepted by my own church. I began attending various churches of differing denominations before I chose one. I can't imagine the psychological pain I would have if I was made to believe that Catholicism was the only acceptable form of worship and I no longer fit in. I didn't like the fact that most churches would preach about the evils of drinking alcohol yet I remember when I worked at a Southern Baptist church one particular night running into one of the deacons buying beer before a football game. He was obviously embarrassed to see me. And he should have been. He was one of the people in the church that was so verbal against drinking. I really didn't care if he liked beer or not but just my presence caused him shame. I do not believe that drinking a beer will send you straight to hell.

I have met lots of people who believe you are not a Christian unless you meet certain criteria. Like abstinence from alcohol and never going through a divorce. There are man's laws and there are God's laws and they are not always the same. A lot of people in the South believe that unless you are "born again" and have been "saved", you are not eligible for the kingdom of heaven. Personally, I had a "saving" experience when I was a teenager. But I do not believe it is necessary. It burns me up to think about it, but as strongly as I feel anger towards people who kill others and molest children, I know that God loves them too. I also know people who are not "born again" that are wonderful Christians and I believe have a place in heaven.

I can tell you that I was "saved" after meeting a group of girls who came to the beach one summer with a Christian missions group. I made some wonderful friends and became very close to the Lord that summer but when they left to go back to school, all my Christian support group was gone and it was tough living in a resort town to keep the faith. I grew up in a party town and there were temptations all over the place. I kept getting myself into these terrible situations and I didn't seem to understand why bad things were happening to me all the time.

I can honestly say that I have experienced personally what I believe to be everything bad that can happen to a young woman except murder. Let me just leave it at that because it would take too much space to go into but I believe everything we go through in our lives affects us in some way. Whether we are destined to do things, or do them out of our own free will, I have trouble deciding. I do know that God is always there for us if we will just allow Him in our lives. Saying a prayer inviting God into our lives is a good first step but I believe it requires a whole lot more than that to be able to call yourself a Christian.

I have noticed that the people who seem to need Him the most are the ones that try so hard to fight against it or either shelter themselves inside church walls and never explore their own behavior. Some people who claim to be Christians live their whole lives without gaining any insight into their own personalities. Even though I was "saved" earlier in my life, I ended up then in more trouble and much farther away from having a personal relationship with Christ than many years later, when I was simply living my life to the best of my abilities without a group of Christian friends that I hung out with.

How does all this relate to cancer? When you are diagnosed is not the best time to assess your faith but it is a good time. I think it would do us all good to think about our own mortality and make plans for the inevitable. We all will die one day. But we refuse to accept it. We are in denial about death. We work hard and neglect our families and our bodies to earn the almighty dollar so that we can buy material pleasures. The thought of death and losing everything you own, your prestige and your "standing" is horrifying to most of us. I think most people spend their whole lives chasing after pleasures that they think will make them happy when in the end there is only death and you can't take them with you. When you are diagnosed with a major illness you think a lot about death. If you are like I was then you have less faith in medicine than you do in spiritual healing. People begin to talk to you a lot about God when you have a life threatening illness. If you are uncomfortable with that now, then you'd better get ready because it's coming. Another thing I have learned is that when you allow yourself to be open to the blessings of living a good life and begin giving of yourself with no expectation of anything in return is when you truly begin receiving miracles, either as a reward for your trust, or by grace itself.

Additionally, our faith can allow us to feel like all things we experience are ordained by God and that He will not allow us to suffer any more than we can deal with. If we are in an environment around other believers they can offer us support and prayer. They can also be a source of inspiration and encouragement. Just for the record, I have been associated with people who are supposedly "born again" that have hurt me very deeply with the intention of doing so. I have also seen devout, hard working church leaders in states of anger and rage so terrible that you would say it was evil.

The church I worked in fired their pastor after spreading nasty rumors all because he believed in allowing members from different ethnic groups. Saying a prayer of acceptance to Jesus did not change their personalities. I would prefer to be surrounded by people that I feel care about me and have a spirit of genuine kindness regardless of their faith, than the people who profess to be Christians but pick and choose who they are going to love and accept. In my experience, certain individuals have rules that don't apply to everyone, only the people that are in their circle of influence. When you look closely at their lives they are as far from understanding the teachings of Christ as I am from understanding rocket science.

Write down your reaction to my beliefs on religion. What do you believe? Do you practice your religion?

Relaxation

Studies have been done for many years on the effects of stress as it relates to disease. For many people who have had cancer, the diagnosis was preceded by a period of intense stress. Life stressors can come in many forms, both good and bad. Take a wedding for example. It is a joyous occasion yet very stressful. Same with a move to another town, or the transfer of a job or school, etc. Bad stressors of course are things like divorce, death of a loved one, unemployment, car troubles, strained relationships, bills, etc.

Take a look at the stressors in your life. It was apparent to me that just before I was diagnosed with cancer I had suffered marital problems and went through a legal separation. Right before the cancer was again discovered in my body I had finished two years of graduate school, bought a house, and started working a new job. Both times I had tremendous stress in my life (good and bad) just before I found out I had cancer.

When I first discovered all the ways that I could assist my body in battling cancer I was overcome with guilt. I felt like this information had been out there previously and if I would have only paid attention maybe I would not have gotten this disease. I had to learn through meditation and prayer that getting cancer was not my fault. Sure, I could have done a lot of things to help prevent the disease, but I came to believe there was a good reason for my having it.

Having cancer taught me to have faith. It taught me to not waste my life. It taught me patience and trust. It also helped me realize that I needed to learn forgiveness. It got me off my rear and into gear to accomplish some dreams that I had always had. I became a kinder soul.

It could very well be that there is a life lesson for you to learn through the experience. You might die. But there may be a lot of wonderful memories you can make now before you die. You may be able to help your body fight long enough to extend your life so that you can accomplish some things. You may yet receive complete healing and never have to worry about cancer again. Whatever way things turn out, please don't blame yourself. You are not the only one in control. There are forces much greater than you at work and you can be guided by this and work with it for greater good. Do what you can to take control of the things that you truly have control of. Don't try to struggle constantly against situations that are not under your power. Don't hate yourself because of your disease. Realize your vulnerability and do what you can to make your live better with a spirit of humility, following the direction in which your cancer experience takes you.

The Serenity Prayer is one of my favorite Christian prayers. It goes, "*God grant me the serenity to accept the things I cannot change, courage to change the things I can, and the wisdom to know the difference*". Serenity, acceptance, courage and wisdom are not bad lessons to learn in life. If it takes having cancer to learn these virtues, then so be it.

Do what you can to give your body a chance to heal. But if things don't go the way you would like for them to, then realize there is a reason for your suffering and try to learn from it. That is what life is all about, learning from our sufferings. Be an example to others. Show them that you can be victorious in all things, no matter what they are. When I told people around me that the doctors said I was terminal, I received many affirmations of my worth! People that had never seemed to have any affection for me suddenly began telling me they loved me. I had numerous people tell me that they admired me and I was an inspiration to them. Some of my friends explained how I had influenced their lives and thanked me for all the things they learned from me. It was awesome. I felt loved and worthwhile. If I had not had cancer, this would not have happened. I consider it a blessing. Having a life-threatening disease is a learning experience. It can teach you how to be real. Discover what truly makes you happy. Find peace in your life. Learn how to relax and just live. See the beauty of the world around you and let go of the forces that drive you to live a life full of stress. Give yourself a break.

Hopefully one thing you will learn to do if you are not doing it already is to be good to yourself. Following are some suggestions for doing so. It was important to me to weed out as many stressors in my life as I could and so I had to learn techniques for doing this. Let the housecleaning go for a change. Don't worry about the laundry or the shopping. It will get done. Don't let the opinions of others push you into doing things that you don't want to do. Eliminate pressure by not answering your phone! Don't feel forced to participate in activities if you would rather do something else. Your children will remember you for the precious times they spent singing, laughing, or talking with you, walking with you holding their hands, not your presence in the bleachers during basketball games or you reading a book outside, waiting for ballet to be over. Re-examine your priorities and re-order your life. Just relax today. Be kind to yourself –don't depend on others for that because you may be disappointed.

How can you re-order your priorities so that you have "me time"?

Yoga

I gave yoga a category of its own because I think it deserves it. It provides simple movements, along with the difficult ones that you can do gently at a low level if you don't have a lot of mobility. It is a wonderful way to de-stress before a bath at the end of the day. It can set up a mood for you of meditation and relaxation that is conducive to prayer, visualization, or simply going to sleep.

Have you ever tried yoga? Can you get a yoga video?

Laughter

My husband will go to the video store once a week and pick up the latest comedies for us to watch. We make popcorn and enjoy the time we have together. Have you ever laughed so hard your sides ache? It's difficult to be concerned about dying when you are rolling in laughter. *Laughter has been proven scientifically to assist healing!* There was a while that I was homebound that I did nothing but watch detective shows where people were committing crimes and homicide was the main theme. During that time, I felt down after watching TV all day. I felt like my life had no purpose. I was addicted to these shows that ruined my mood and my chances of having a good, productive day.

How many times per day do you laugh?

Music

Go to the movies and notice how the music sets the tone for certain scenes. Close your eyes and even though you cannot see you know still when it is time for a romantic moment versus a scary one. I don't think I could survive without music. There is one song on a CD that I have that I play almost every morning because it puts me in a good mood. I call it "my happy song". It is upbeat and cheerful. You can choose music to match your mood too. Try doing yoga to classical music, or aerobics to dance music. Experiment with sounds of nature combined with music and do your visualization exercise with that in the background. We also have a tendency to get angry and impatient when listening to certain types of music, so choose selections that only make you feel good.

Do you ever listen to music that makes you feel good? Write the names of the songs down.

Candles

I love candles! They give such a warm, natural light that is soothing and the wax is fragrant too. I light candles all the time in my home because they provide a comforting, meditative mood.

Light a candle right now.

Aromatherapy

This has gotten a lot of attention in recent years. The scents of certain botanicals are especially pleasing in candles, lotions, bubble baths, and room sprays. There is a belief that the smell of certain herbs and botanicals actually has healing properties. Different aromas are used for different things, like lavender and chamomile for calming and citrus fruits and ginger for energizing.

Notice the next time you smell a good scent how it makes you feel. What is it? Write it down.

Bubble baths

Do I need to say anything about this? Although I would not recommend it when you are over 250 lbs. because you might get stuck in the tub as I did! I have a friend who calls me when she takes a bath because that is when she has enough quiet time to think.

Set aside time to take a bubble bath tonight.

Hot tubs

My mother-in-law has one of these in her sun room. If you have access to one, by all means take advantage of it.

Is there a hot tub nearby that you can use? What about a Jacuzzi tub? Foot massager with pulsing water?

Massages

Breast cancer patients are advised not to have a deep tissue massage because it stimulates lymph flow and in some cases, it is suspected to cause the cancer to spread. Having your back and shoulders rubbed by a loved one though is wonderful.

Have you ever had a professional massage? Tell your loved ones that they can buy you one as a gift the next time they ask you if there is anything they can do!

Meditation

Meditation is an art. The more you practice, the better you become with it. You lie down in the most comfortable position you can be in. I would suggest lying in bed or on the floor on your back with no pillow and your body straight with your arms at your sides but I know a lot of people cannot lie this way. The most important thing is that you are comfortable. You clear your mind of all its clutter. This was very difficult for me to learn to do but if you use visualization first, it usually helps. Then you focus on one small area of your body at a time, beginning with your toes. Imaging that they are very heavy, like they are covered in lead. Release all the tensions you can. Slowly work your way up your body until you get to your face. The worst area for me is my mouth. I want to hold it closed but the most relaxed position for your mouth is slightly open. Just lie there until you feel your body melt away. *You will get to the point that you can literally feel like you have stepped out of your physical body.* This is when you just allow peaceful feelings to flow through you and I have found that my most profound "visions" or "messages" come to me after I do this.

That reminds me to tell you to always keep a journal and a pen next to you bed. A lot of times we experience dreams or images that we will not remember in the morning and it is fascinating to write these down immediately after they happen and then go through in the morning, analyzing them. My best inspirations and ideas come to me at these times.

There have been times in my life when I felt hurt or insulted by others and my immediate response was to become angry and want revenge. I began burying my nose in the Bible during these times and finding a scripture passage there that really summed up my situation. I would write the passage down, get to a quiet, dimly lit place, and begin my meditation by repeating this scripture over and over. Rather than picturing in my mind how satisfied I would feel slapping someone in the face, I began picturing myself in the armor of God, covered in light, surrounded by peace and serenity where nothing could rattle me or cause me to feel bad thoughts.

It is also a way to vent those feelings of frustration that you inevitably feel towards your partner in a way that is not confrontational. Sometimes our anger controls us and we say things we don't really mean. Once you've said it aloud, you cannot take it back. There are some things that once you've said them, you've crossed a line that is hard to undo. Things like "I hate you" and "Why don't we get a divorce" are things like this. I think it is much better to write these feelings down and that way you can "edit" it before you say it.

Have you ever meditated? After you do, write down the way it made you feel and/or the thoughts you had afterwards.

Visualization

These are mental exercises, similar to self-hypnosis. You make your own movies inside your head and you watch them play out. In the beginning it is hard to hold onto an image because you may get so relaxed that you fall asleep, But in time this will become second nature to you. *Visualization and positive imagery are proven to be helpful to cancer victims in reducing pain and in some cases, the actual growth of cancer in the body has been reversed.* Coincidence? I told you I don't believe in those anymore. I have exercises that I do when the house is quiet, usually at bedtime. I will share with you some examples that I use.

Imagine you are on a calm beach or a safe place of your choosing. In my visualization, I approach the beach from an old weather-worn cabana. I watch my feet as I step down slowly one step at a time to the sand. I walk across the warm, white sand and find a lounge chair shaded by an umbrella. I recline in the chair and begin to get relaxed, listening to the waves and the gulls and feeling the warm breeze pass over my skin. The air is filled with smells: the salt from the ocean and the smell of sea foam, the woody scent of sea oats, and the sweet odor of seaweed that has washed up on the shore. A tiny hole in the center of the umbrella lets in a stream of light that begins to warm my head. I imagine it is healing light from God. The light moves slowly over my entire body and as it does it heals every inch of my being. When it is finished, I can either fall asleep or get up refreshed.

I am lying in a meadow, surrounded by tall grasses and wildflowers. The sun shines warm on my face and I am breathing in fresh air that is perfumed with the scents of nature all around me. I lift my arms to the sky in a gesture that signifies I am willing to accept God's blessings. Flowers begin falling from the clouds and land in the space between my arms, like they are forming a vessel. God sends me peace and love, good health and comfort. I know that whatever my needs are He will provide and worry has no place in my life.

I lie there and accept as many blessings as he gives and then I fold my arms against my body, allowing the blessings to become part of me, melding with my soul. I stand up and give thanks for the blessings I have just received. Every time I offer a word of encouragement to another, or do something inherently good I know that I am investing in the blessings I will receive the next time.

I am stressed by things that seem to be out of control in my life. I sit down and visualize all of the things that are causing me stress as tangible objects. I put them on one side. Then the things that are good in my life I put on the other side. One by one, I stuff the bad things in black balloons. These are things like bills, people I have issues with, the house, car, cancer cells, little red balls of anger, etc. One by one I stuff the good things in the white balloons. These are my children, my husband, all the people in my life I care for, white balls of happiness, clean cells, etc. Then I collect all the balloons and take them outside. I climb to the top of a high peak and let them go, one by one, looking to see what they are as I release them towards heaven. The black balloons will be given special attention to be straightened out and the white balloons will be blessed and protected. I watch them float away, one by one until they are all gone. I have occasionally envisioned my parents at the other end (they are both deceased) gathering up the balloons in Heaven and personally delivering them to the Almighty.

Again, I am at the beach (you may want to be in a forest or near a waterfall, on snowy mountains or in the country. Just use whatever you think your “happy place” is). I am wearing a flowing white cotton dress and straw hat. My hair is floating in the breeze and it is long and beautiful. I am holding a wooden box, filled with all the emotions that I have trouble dealing with or specific problems that I am having. I am standing in the shallow water with the waves washing over my feet. I set the box down in the water and let the ocean take it away. Each successive wave pulls it further out to see and I watch it blend with horizon until I can no longer see it and I am sure it is gone.

There is a war going on inside my body. It is the good forces against the bad and of course the good guys are in white. The bad guys are in black and they are on horseback brandishing weapons and wearing heavy armor, like in the dark ages. They are fighting with swords and bows, etc. The white army is my immune system, mainly white blood cells. The black army is cancer and of course I try to always see this one through to the end with the black army being totally defeated.

This is a silly image that I saw on TV one night and couldn't get out of my head. It was a face, a combination that looked like part Pac-man and part Frankenstein. It moves rapidly and is continuously chomping at anything in its path with razor sharp teeth. I unleash it on my tumors until it devours all of them and there is nothing left.

Finally, I will share a strange one with you. Because I was diagnosed when I was young, my hair was dark and had no gray. I would often catch myself wondering what I would look like in a coffin. I know, it's morbid but I have a vivid imagination. I began paying close attention to the woman in the coffin and realizing that she was old, with gray hair and wrinkles. I envisioned myself dead finally at around 80 years old.

Try one of these exercises tonight when you go to bed.

Psychotherapy

Why do you think Euthanasia exists? Because people are afraid of pain. If their pet is in pain and suffering, putting them down is always an option. People will seek out assisted death if they are in a lot of pain, commit suicide, self-medicate with alcohol or drugs, or lose their quality of life because they are taking pain meds all the time. We give fear control over our lives. At the dentist's office one day I was waiting in the exam room to be seen and a child was next door having her teeth cleaned. She was terrified and screamed every time an instrument was brought near her mouth. Her fears had taken over. She would cry out in pain before her teeth were even touched.

We allow our fears to force us into making decisions and acting in a way that is unnatural to us. Our minds have enormous power. They can also be used as incredible tools to help us. We can learn to adjust our thinking to always be open to the realm of possibilities and not be guided by fear. I believe very strongly in the power of the human psyche or I would not have chosen therapy as a career. And I am sure that my mental state had a lot to do with whether I was in a state of decline or not. One day I asked my oncologist, "Am I a candidate for anti-depressants?" and he replied, "Every patient I have is a candidate for anti-depressants."

We accumulate issues or "baggage" as some people put it, just from innocently living our lives. Things happen to us that we are ashamed of, make us angry, or encourage us to believe that we are cursed or unlucky. We are victimized by life circumstances without our permission and sometimes without our knowledge. This is aside from the fact that we sometimes make bad choices. Making mistakes is part of being human. It is how we learn. Watch a baby and how it tests its limits time and again, until it is sure of its boundaries. It is trying to learn by correcting its mistakes. But some mistakes we make cause us to feel regret and guilt.

Therapy can help us deal with negative feelings and unlock memories that have been pushed so far into our subconscious mind that we have difficulty recalling them with accuracy. We all have "secrets" that we wouldn't dare share with the outside world for fear of being criticized, shunned, or seen as less than "normal". Finding a good therapist I think is an essential part of our modern lives. There is so much chaos in the world we live in that it is very confusing just to live and difficult sometimes to feel like you belong.

Nowadays therapy is much more accepted than it used to be. At one time, to admit you were seeing a therapist was like saying you were defective. Now it is fashionable. It has almost become a status symbol. If the subject of therapy is brought up at a social function, it is amazing how many people you learn have been going to a therapist for years and will admit it and even recommend it. Some people will run to their therapist every time they break a fingernail and yet others wouldn't see a counselor even if they were married to a psychopath. There are people who are so chained by their emotions that they don't dare take a closer look because they are afraid of what they may find. But I am telling you, as a cancer patient, you need therapy.

Therapy has been termed the "talking cure" and this is so true. All of our experiences are stored in our subconscious minds and tapping into them allows them to begin to escape. Have you ever tried to remember someone's name and couldn't and then days later it just popped into your head? Why does this happen? When we pose a question to our subconscious mind where our memories are stored, the brain begins searching the database. We are not aware of all the work our brain does but eventually it will open the right compartment where that information we seek is stored and produce it for us. We have to make a conscious effort to begin this process. Some memories are stored away so far back into the corner recesses of our minds that they take longer to get to the front where they can be retrieved. Sometimes memories are like pieces of a jigsaw puzzle and often we can find answers to our problems by putting the pieces together and solving the puzzle. Therapy is a good place to start.

We all need someone to talk to. The reason I started this book initially is because I started writing down my feelings and experiences because I was so alone. I needed to express myself and there was no one to talk to. My mother was too sick, and my sister and my best friends were long distance (although there were some hefty phone bills in those days) so I sought out group therapy for cancer patients. It turned out that didn't work for me. The woman who was leading the group had never had cancer and besides, she had recently had a breast enlargement and enjoyed showing them off. That offended me. Also, there was one "submarine" in the group. This is what my profession calls a person in a group that wants to bring everybody down. I went once and that was enough.

I later found a therapist that I loved. She taught me a lot about taking care of myself. I learned that it was okay if sometimes I felt angry or frustrated or pitied myself. After all, I was human and these are human emotions. I had a lot of issues with my divorce and I believe therapy helped me a great deal with that. When I went to grad school, exploring my inner self and trying to gain insight into my own behavior was a requirement of all my classes in various forms. Because I came from a highly dysfunctional family, I had a lot of work to do. On one assignment, the introspection was much too deep for me at the time and I wrote an entire paper on my anger at going through all this emotion without having the therapeutic process to help me put myself back together afterwards. Instead of failing me on the spot, my professor realized that I was just going through the process of recognizing my own human inadequacies and he didn't penalize me.

It was extremely hard at times and I would never say I know the best way to handle things, but I learned that my values are my own and I only have to go by those in order to get along in life. You cannot please everyone so you have to decide who your friends will be and who you want to please.

We don't get to choose our families and some of us are disappointed in the environment in which we were born. If those relationships are causing us pain, we don't have to keep going back for more punishment. I learned that it is okay if you're not pleased with your family of origin. Just simply surround yourself with people that are respectful of your feelings and affirm your worth. You don't have to have "Norman Rockwell" holidays to feel loved and worthwhile. I don't think I have ever even met a single "Norman Rockwell" family in my lifetime.

I offer counseling online via email. If you are interested in therapy or would just simply like to have someone that you can express yourself with, go to www.onlinecounselor.info and email me. This is a service for anyone, not just people who have experienced cancer.

What is your experience with psychotherapy? Find a therapist or support group in your area this week. Call and make an appointment or reserve your place in the group and make a commitment.

Positive affirmations

These are statements that you make to yourself which affirm a positive outcome. They are similar to positive visualizations. I would mutter them to myself or write them down multiple times. Say them with conviction and you will start to believe them! Example: "I am being healed. The cancer in my body is dying. I feel good and I am getting well. I have more energy than ever. I will be alive for a long time."

I used to say, "my head is killing me," instead of "my head hurts." Makes me wonder how my body responded to such negativity. Not only was I feeding myself negativity, but I constantly listened to significant others criticizing me. I don't think our subconscious minds can distinguish between truth and lies. If you raise a child up in an abusive and negligent home, that child grows up to believe that violence is the only solution to problems and that he is worthless. *The negative statements we hear to be the truth can be very damaging.* If someone tells you when you are going to die, dismiss the statement immediately. It is based on averages and in my opinion, there's no such thing. Nobody knows how long you will live. To assume that they have the omnipotent knowledge of the number of your days on earth is absurd and egotistical. I believe that because God is my Creator, only He knows how long I will live and by not revealing it to me he is allowing me to live on faith.

There are a lot of wonderful books available on positive affirmations. Some are written like devotionals, where you have a concept to focus on each day. I would definitely get my hands on a copy to use for my healing. Some have a spiritual lean and some are just feel good books but no matter which kind you end up with, they are great tools. I am writing down the affirmations that I use and one day I may have it published. In the meantime, think of the topics that you need the most help with and write your own statements of affirmation that address your weaknesses. Say this to yourself every day in a tone of authority and belief. Write affirmations on index cards and keep them in a file box. Every day take one out and carry it with you. Keep it in your pocket and you have access to it whether you are at work, in the grocery store, driving in the car and stuck in traffic, etc.

Three positive affirmations I can use now are:

Goal setting

I believe this is one of the most important things that we can do in order to take care of ourselves. We all have dreams and goals and I had the experience of putting all of mine on the back burner while I focused on the goals of other people. When I started having kids, it was easy to allow my role as their mother to take over my life and somehow I went from being an intelligent, talented and attractive woman with ambition and aspirations to being someone else's wife or mother and nothing else. Please don't misunderstand me. I loved being married and having kids and being part of a family but I despised losing myself along the way. I am not blaming or making excuses. It was my choice.

I think had I been diagnosed while I was still married to the children's father I would have died then. The way I felt was that I had lost my own identity. It was a very negative, unloving atmosphere. I never felt emotionally supported by my spouse. He would criticize me just as easily as he would a stranger. My life had no meaning then, no purpose. We were trying to keep up with the Jones's and it was at a breakneck speed. He was constantly overspending. His motto was, "why should I do it when I can pay to have someone else do it?" We ate out just about every night. Not fast food, but full course meals in a sit-down restaurant. We would go out to eat so often that we were on a first name basis with most restaurant owners. We also had a housekeeper who did laundry and ironing, someone to tend to the yard, babysitters, employees who would wash the cars and cook food for us at the restaurant he ran, and so forth. I was totally stressed out by the demands I put upon myself in order to feel like I was an acceptable member of society.

When I was on my own, however, things changed. I no longer had the income to compete in the rat race and my priorities started changing. I began to renew interests that I had not even given thought to in many years. One day I thought about dying and what my funeral would be like. I wondered if anyone would attend. The more I thought about that, the angrier I became because at one time I had lots of genuine friends but along the way we became estranged, one by one. I knew that it wasn't like me to not have friends and other people in my life. I began to reach out to others more and try to make friends with people wherever I went. I made it my mission to benefit the lives of others.

Because I felt like I had neglected myself all that time, I thought it was important to make some goals and work towards them. This is when I enrolled in graduate school. Now let me say that graduate school was a lofty goal and the only reason I was able to do that was because I wasn't working and was going through treatment instead. A goal is best when it is small. For example: When I was told in September that I would only live for two months, I hopped down from the exam table in my doctor's office shaking my head saying, "No, that is not enough time". My son's birthday was in November and I didn't want him to always associate that time with my death instead of his birth. I simply asked God to let me live at least until after that. Then it was Thanksgiving. Soon it would be Christmas, then New Year's. Both my daughter and my sister had birthdays in February so it couldn't be then either! Then there was St. Patrick's Day (my son's namesake which we always celebrated), Mother's day, my birthday, Dill's birthday, etc. You see the pattern. Every time I jumped one goal hurdle, there was another one in front of me. I felt like some people in my family needed me and I think that helped me live!

I have never been content just sitting around the house. I need to be busy. Since I could no longer work, I began volunteering for an agency that was near and dear to my heart-counseling victims of domestic violence. I couldn't do clerical work or provide transportation for them but I could talk on the phone and so that is what I started doing. Answering their crisis calls. *There is nothing better to take your mind off your own problems than to talk to others who are in crisis*. It doesn't matter how bad your situation is, seeing others in pain is a grounding experience. It always keeps me real. It is easy to get into a rut and feel sorry for yourself because you cannot do things like other people you know, and you can no longer keep up with the Joneses, etc. But I found that just as often as you notice the grass may be a little greener on the other side of the fence, you come in contact with someone whose needs you cannot even comprehend they are so great. These are the times that I thank God for taking care of me and allowing us to provide for our family.

A debilitating disease like the one I had causes you to change your perspective. When I no longer fit into my "peer" group because I couldn't wear my fashionable clothes, had no career, couldn't participate in activities anymore, couldn't drive, became wheelchair bound, lost my hair, etc., my old constructs began to fade away. At one time, I would see someone wearing a pair of shoes I thought was really cute and I would make it a point to find some like that. Or I might see a nice hairstyle on someone else and tell my stylist to copy it on me. Once my perspective began to change, so did my goals. I no longer had the desire to be stylish and fashionable. It would have been nice, but it was no longer my only motivation in life. Living my life one day at a time, being alive for my family, and doing what I could in the time that I had left to help others in need became my focus.

Write down your 1 week, 1 month, 3 month, 6 month, 1 year, 5 year, 10 year goals:

Hobbies

This is another way to attack boredom. I started trying to crochet again when I had to resign from my job. I made my kids scarves and let them pick the colors. I even made my daughter's doll a scarf and it was fun. Besides, I was giving them something that I had created and even my ten-year-old son realized the significance of that. He said to me, "I'll always have this scarf you made for me, even when you are gone". The day after I was told I was terminal, my sister and I went shopping. I wanted to buy the kids stuff that they could remember me by. I bought each of them a small chest, photo albums, address books, and journals. I bought my son some tools and my daughter some cosmetic cases. Here was my logic: I would fill the photo albums with pictures we had taken together. I would record addresses of my extended family and friends in case when they were older they wanted to ask others about me if I was gone. I wrote in the journals what each of them meant to me and what I thought their individual strengths were. I left the remaining pages blank and wrote each of them a note to encourage them to write to me if I was gone and they wanted to talk to me. The tools and cosmetic cases were things that I thought would last a long time and I put all of these things in their chests for them to have after I die. I also started compiling a cookbook of my mother's recipes and my recipes and documented a little story about each one. *I was preparing a "legacy" for them.*

Other things I think are good ideas are to write a story together, color together, make a quilt, write poetry, paint, etc. One of the things that I do that gives me a lot of pleasure is grow roses. I love gardening. There is something about plunging your hands into the Earth and watching a living thing grow that really gives you a sense of satisfaction. My son looks for the prettiest blooms in the rose bushes and cuts it for me. Whenever I see him coming in with a rose for me it makes my heart smile. I have saved them all and made potpourri out of them or dried them upside down in my kitchen window. My daughter always draws a picture for me to hang on the refrigerator door. I spend time with her teaching her how to draw and this is how she rewards me. They are both really proud of themselves when they do something that pleases me. Share something tangible with your loved ones so that they have something to remember you by when you are gone.

Write down things hobbies you would be interested in pursuing immediately:

Journaling

The first time I heard this term was my first experience in therapy. I had at various times in my life written in a diary, but I would always go back and read through what I had written and be embarrassed at myself and destroy it. That is, until that fateful day when I realized I might have cancer. Then every moment of my life mattered, embarrassing or not.

Go out and buy yourself a journal or just use a spiral-bound notebook or your computer. Start your journal today with an entry about how you found out you had cancer and what your feelings were.

This is my journal beginning with the day I began to explore the meaning of my existence. At first I called it my "cancer diary" on my computer but it didn't take long for me to realize that every time I wrote in it, I was writing in a document about a disease, not a life. So I renamed it my "life diary". It summarized my thoughts and feelings, as well as both the ordinary and extraordinary events of my days following the discovery of cancer in my body. Even though it is highly personal, I want to share it with you. If anyone who shares this journey is somehow touched or made better by the experience then it has been well worth it. If I offend anyone involved by revealing intimate details, I apologize. I changed names where I thought it was appropriate. I cannot leave anything else out because the picture would not be complete and accurate. These are the reflections of my soul, poured out in black text on white paper…honest and unpretentious. This is me.

May 13, 2000

I had not been awake very long, contemplating my circumstances and life in general. I stretched out, yawning, with both arms up and turning my head side to side, listening for my neck to crack when I noticed the swelling. It wasn't the first time I had seen it. I had thought several times before in previous weeks, perhaps months that my left underarm was puffy but this day it seemed worse. I ran my fingers over the bulge and began pressing into the surrounding area, searching for some kind of clue. When I felt the knot under my chest muscle, I suddenly got dizzy. "No, no it can't be," I thought silently.

My first thoughts turned to my mother, who was waiting to hear results back on another lump she had discovered in her chest. She had no breasts, having lost one to cancer when I was in the 5th grade in the 70's and the other only 4 years ago. Breast cancer runs in my family. This was my mother's 3rd episode of it, the same wretched disease that had claimed the life of her sister many years before. I was numb.

I remembered going to see a doctor several years ago about a round lump I had felt just under my ribcage. "Aww, it's nothing…just a swollen lymph node…you may have a slight infection somewhere in your body but don't worry about it," she had said. "My God," I thought, "what is happening to me? Could this be related to that discovery? And if it is, just how long have I been walking around with this, not knowing?" (I was told later by a physician that we do not even have lymph nodes there!)

I examined my breasts to the best of my ability and felt nothing more. I avoided talking to anyone that day, going through the motions of my life like a zombie. I planned to call a doctor first thing Monday morning.

May 14

Today is Mother's Day and since it was his week of custody, Jim brought the kids over to visit me. We have been separated for four months. While he was here I decided to tell him about the knot I had found. He just shook his head and had little to say. I was uneasy and nervous. I had trouble looking at him. After a long silence, he came over to me and reached out to hug me. I backed away. He said, "I am only trying to comfort you. You need comforting." I hesitantly put my arms around him and he squeezed me. I began to weep, then sob. I broke the embrace and went into the kitchen. He followed me. He embraced me again, ran his fingers through my hair, tugging my head back and tried to kiss me. I turned my face away. Before he left he snappily said, "Even though you don't love me you know I will be there for you because that is the type of person I am. Just remember that when I am the only one there." I wanted to hit him. In anger, I decided that I would rather go through this alone than have him there.

May 17

I made an appointment with the Obstetrician who had delivered my son seven years ago. He is a good doctor with a great reputation in town. He is serious and matter-of-fact, as opposed to his partner, who is bubbly and witty. Of the two doctors, I prefer the latter most times but today was different. I needed cold hard facts delivered by someone who would be blunt and to the point.

As I waited in the lobby I imagined what would happen when it came time to pay for my visit. My husband had agreed to keep me on his family health insurance policy throughout our legal separation. I knew that this doctor was not an accepted medical provider for the insurance company but I just assumed I could get a receipt and file it myself. I hoped this would work.

A new father sat on the sofa across from me with his premature baby girl. He cuddled her and kissed her and teased her lips with a bottle. She instinctively accepted and began sucking. My mind turned to my little girl. She had been born five years ago and the day I left the hospital with her was the last time I had seen my doctors. I had not had a pap smear since. I was to have a mammogram the year I turned 35 but had procrastinated. In ten days I would be 37. The nurse interrupted my thoughts by calling me back to the exam room.

"When did you discover this lump?" Dr. Pierce asked. "Sunday," I answered. He couldn't seem to find it or at least wasn't concerned. He concentrated on my breasts. "Were you going to tell me about this one?" he asked. In disbelief I bolted upright on the table. He eased me back down and placed my hand over my left breast. It felt like the shape and size of a peach pit. The room grew dark. "Get Sandra, I want an ultrasound," he ordered the nurse. It seemed like they were talking and moving in slow motion.

Sandra had accurately predicted the sex of both my children in previous years. She was kind and gentle and had a sweet disposition. As I lay on the table, I remembered her telling me back then how difficult her job could be when instead of preparing her patients for wallpaper, she sometimes had to prepare them for the baby's funeral. I wanted to cry.

The doctor came in and watched the monitor as she slid the apparatus over my slimy breast. "That's it right there and it's solid." She turned to him and nodded. He instructed me to get dressed and meet him in his study.

"This is a picture of the breast. The mass you have is located here. It is not a cyst because it is solid. It could be a fibroid tumor, which would be benign. I do not see any indications of cancer but you need to see a surgeon and have a biopsy." I asked for a recommendation. He made a phone call. I sat there quietly and still but my mind was racing. I seldom got sick. I didn't take medication. I had never had as much as a broken bone, not to mention surgery.

I paid fifty dollars towards the bill and asked to pay the rest later. It was fifty dollars I did not have. Since I had left my husband on New Years Day, I had struggled to make ends meet. There had been weeks that I ate only toast and coffee because money was so scarce. I would get my meager paychecks every Friday and sit down at the dining table, going over my bills again and again, as if something would magically happen and I would figure out a way to pay them all. This could get really bad.

May 22

I had some conversations with Jim about the insurance situation. He assured me everything was fine, but he was not convincing. Something in the way he stammered around the issue bothered me. I don't think he really knew whether I had insurance or not and the worst part is, I don't think he even considered how serious an issue it could be. But he does now.

When I got to the surgeon's office, the receptionist took my insurance card and made a call to the company to verify coverage. The office was cold, like a meat locker. I was trembling and wringing my hands in a feeble effort to try and warm my fingers. She was on the phone for what seemed like an eternity. I saw the look on her face before she said anything. When she covered the phone receiver with her hand, I knew what she was going to tell me. "Your insurance was cancelled in April. I'm sorry. This could be very expensive."

I felt like I had strong hands around my neck, choking me. The tears welled up instantly, uncontrollably. "Please give me my card back and cancel my appointment. I'm sorry for the inconvenience." The tears hit the floor before I ever got out of the office. By the time I got to my car, I was running like a scared animal. Panic. I was tired of waiting to find out what was wrong with me. I was tired of worrying about money. I was tired of the way the fear was controlling me. I wanted out.

As I reached for the car door to shut it, I saw him approaching through the blur of tears. He grabbed the door so I couldn't close it and knelt down on the pavement. "Where are you going?" he asked me. "I'm leaving!" I managed to mutter between sobs. He held out his hand. I reluctantly shook it. "I'm Dr. Elvis. Why did you come to see me today?" I told him I had a lump in my breast. He told me to come back inside and he would examine me at no charge. In disbelief I followed him to the exam room, past the patients waiting, past the woman on the phone, past the nurses.

I cried like a baby as I struggled to answer his questions about my family history. He asked them while examining me. Afterwards, he put his hand on my knee and tried to comfort me. He ordered a mammogram for the next day. He wanted to help me get something done soon. He knew I needed answers. I left his office feeling like I had encountered an angel. As I drove to my mother's house, the tears continued to pour in a steady stream down my face. "Thank you God," I repeated like a mantra. When I told my mother what happened, she also cried. "God is looking out for you Betty," she said. "He is in control. Don't forget that for a moment." She handed me a tranquilizer to take when I got home. "Go to sleep tonight and don't worry. You can win this."

That night I kissed my father's picture and asked him to help me. He passed away 5 years ago. He had a massive heart attack just days after completing his radiation for the cancer on his vocal chords. He survived on life support in intensive care for 29 excruciating days and then died 11 days before Christmas. I hated going to that hospital. I said I would never go there again. I didn't know that I would soon have surgery in the very same place.

The next morning I had work to do. I was going to get to the bottom of the insurance problem and someone would have hell to pay. I was angry. I was confrontational. After several conversations over the phone with the insurance company and with my lawyer, I was assured that my expenses would be covered if I chose to go to the physician that participated in the insurance plan. With a sigh I asked whom to go to. When I heard the name of my father's physician, I cried again. I thought the world of him. I called and cancelled the mammogram ordered by Dr. Elvis and made an appointment for one the next day at the other hospital. Dr. Pollard was on vacation and wouldn't return until the following Monday but I got an appointment for Wednesday after he got back. My results would go to him.

<u>May 24</u>

I put on my wedding band in the morning for the first time in a long time. I had decided that I would no longer worry about the medical bills. Without insurance, my husband would be responsible for them and I would simply let him handle it. Today I would present myself as Mrs. Henson. I knew his social security number from memory and I would use it for billing purposes if I had to. I arrived at the radiology center in a good mood. I felt relieved that I was finally going to be tested.

In the waiting room, I read magazines about love and sex and growing old. I wondered if I would ever love again, ever have sex again, and if I would grow old. I met a woman who chatted with me while she waited for X-Rays. She talked about her aunt who had recently died from cancer. I asked who her doctor was. She said it had been Dr. Elvis. I told her the story about my encounter with him. She beamed. "Sounds like a miracle to me," she commented. I thought of my mother's words and secretly thanked God.

The mammography technician was a plump, young, attractive girl with long beautiful red hair. She stuck adhesive "markers" on my breast in the vicinity of the lump and put metallic tape over my nipples. She maneuvered my breasts onto the plates and talked about what a good patient I was. Afterwards, she informed me that the lump was the same density as my breast tissue and could not be detected on the mammogram. She was sending me to sonography.

I lay on the cot in the darkness waiting. The dim light from the computer monitor and the hum of the equipment made me drowsy. I drifted off to sleep just before the door opened. I mused at how much like the other girl this one looked as she squeezed the cold jelly onto my breast. She had difficulty finding the mass and switched her transducer to a more sensitive one. She showed me the image. It looked like black storm clouds, with one particularly nasty looking one in the background. "That's it," she said. She called in her boss. The radiologist viewed the monitor while spilling out his routine words of encouragement about early detection. I felt like I was listening to a TV commercial.

That night I soaked my tired body in a hot bubble bath. My breast was painfully sore. I lit candles in my room and listened to soft music while I sent e-mail letters to my friends to tell them what was going on. When I lay down to go to sleep, I tried to remember how to meditate. I relaxed my body and imagined the bright white light of God's healing searing into my breast. I basked in the warmth of its rays and my body went numb. I felt as though I was floating in the sky. I went to sleep easily and slept soundly until morning.

May 27

My 37th birthday. For the past several years, I spent this particular weekend out of town in my favorite hotel with my husband and children. We would take the kids to the state museum and the zoo on Saturday. We would order room service and drink cocktails in the hotel at night and during the day on Sunday we would shop for antiques. I always looked forward to that little getaway. This weekend I would not be going. I was no longer part of the "family". Jim took the kids without me, which is what I expected. I hoped that they were having fun.

I spent the evening alone in a dark apartment. I pried the cork out of a bottle of wine with a steak knife because I didn't own a corkscrew. I proceeded to drink the entire contents from a coffee mug because I didn't own a wineglass. I chatted on the phone for several hours long distance with my friend Dill. He had become my sounding board, my therapist, my comforter, my cheerleader, my coach. Not only was he a great listener, but he also shared himself with me.

Having his trust and confidence was sacred to me. Even though he lived so far away, I had become very close to him since my separation and this was difficult for people to understand but his friendship was my sustenance. I felt like he was a lifeline for me, keeping me from drowning. I talked to him until I couldn't talk anymore.

He stayed on the phone, sharing the meaningful silence with me in his usual compassionate, caring, and utterly extraordinary manner. He fell asleep on the phone and I listened to his peaceful steady breathing for half an hour before I hung up and went to sleep, too overwhelmed with love and gratitude for Dill to care about cancer and too intoxicated to think about it.

June 2

Every year our town holds a 5K Run on the beach in celebration of summer. Every year I consider entering and every year I regret not doing it. This year that has changed. Although I can hardly walk 5K, I made the decision to enter. I convinced my niece to do it with me and we braved the sand together. My number was 829 and thanks to no parking and a late arrival, she and I were the last numbers out and had to run just to catch up to the pack of walkers! But we did it. It was a small thing in the eyes of some but to me it was the accomplishment of a dream. I am now wearing my trophy T-Shirt and feeling proud. I will do this again.

I cannot remember much else I did this past week other than struggle to endure 40 hours of work. I informed my boss and certain family members and friends of the update in my condition. It was one of the longest weeks of my life. Dill had been planning to come down and visit me soon and was waiting to hear from his job when he could make the trip. I wanted to see him but not under these circumstances. I wanted his visit to be fun and happy. I wanted to be my usual carefree and frivolous self. I tried to stay busy cleaning my apartment and making plans for his arrival.

One night I had a vivid dream. I was standing in front of the bathroom mirror putting on my makeup. I had no hair and no eyebrows. I was penciling in a reddish line where my eyebrows should have been. I put on blue eye shadow and bright red lipstick. I lay down on the floor naked in front of my floral printed sofa, propped up on my elbows, closed my eyes, and leaned my head back. Someone was there taking a picture of me.

When I woke up, I replayed the dream in my head. I wondered what the picture of that would have looked like. Suddenly I remembered a painting I had done in a college watercolor class 15 years earlier and I felt like I was going to faint. I had painted myself as a bald woman with colorful skin, reclining naked. Blood fell from the sky like rain on me and as it touched my body, each drop turned into a flower. I didn't know if that painting still existed but I wanted to find it (by the way, I did find that painting 3 years later and it is printed on the cover of this book if you want to see it)!

June 5

This morning I had trouble waking up my daughter for school. No matter what I did, she would go right back to sleep. I was running late. I worried that she might be sick. I didn't know how I would face another day at work when my mind was elsewhere. I called in and told them my daughter was ill. I lay back down in the bed beside her and stroked her hair. My son joined us. We lay arm in arm, the three of us, talking about love and families and God.

I had the urge to call my mother. We decided I should take her to her appointment that day with Dr. Pollard since I wasn't working. She was going to see if she needed more surgery for her latest breast lump. She called the office to confirm and told them I was taking her. They said to tell me that the doctor would see me too. My mother said, "You see? God is in this." I knew she was right. I felt his presence.

My son stayed in the car and played his hand held computer game while we waited. My mother was called in, then me. My daughter asked why I was there. I told her my arm was hurting and I needed to find out why. She danced around the exam room until my mother emerged and as the doctor came in, I sent her out to stay with her Grandma. I didn't want her to be there.

He felt the lump in my breast and immediately turned his attention to my underarm. I studied his face carefully as he held my arm in the crook of his and massaged my lymph nodes. He looked concerned and uneasy. He squeezed my hand and looked at me over the top of his glasses, with his head bowed and his arms folded. "I cannot be sure", he said. "I am sending you to the hospital tomorrow to have a needle aspiration and then we will know one way or the other." I thanked him for seeing me that day. As I headed out to the car, he pulled my mother aside and whispered, "I want you to be there with her tomorrow."

June 6

I called my mother last night and told her that I wanted to go to the hospital alone. She had trouble understanding this. My mother thrived on tragedy. She was a survivor and had suffered through more pain than any one human being should have to endure. Three encounters with breast cancer, uncontrollable diabetes, emphysema, chronic bronchitis, macular degeneration, cataracts, gall bladder surgery, a pacemaker, and two open-heart surgeries had left her with scars from her ankles to her eyeballs. Every time she cleared a medical hurdle, another loomed ahead. Being sick was her life and I didn't want to inherit that from her. I didn't want to witness the despair she would inevitably feel if she was there, as if she could will to me her same fate.

The lab technician introduced herself as Kristen. I instantly liked her. She described the procedure to me and I warned her that I had a similar test on my thyroid 15 years prior and passed out. She promised she would catch me if I did. I smiled. My blood was drawn and she took me into the office of the pathologist who was a masculine looking young woman with short dark hair, no makeup, and a man's gait, wearing khaki trousers and a button-down shirt. She sat me down in an office chair and Kristen knelt beside me, holding my hand. She inserted a long thin needle strapped to an apparatus that resembled a gun and I flinched. She dug the needle around inside my breast and I squeezed Kristen's hand with all my strength. She expelled the bloody sample onto a slide and said apologetically, "I have to do it again." This time Kristen squeezed first. They said I would know something within the hour and to go to the doctor's office and wait. I got dressed and headed out the door. As I was leaving, Kristen said, "Good luck," and I replied "Thanks, see you later." I felt like I would see her again. I was trembling and my knees were weak as I walked to the car.

Dr. Pollard's receptionist caught my eye as soon as I entered the office and motioned for me to go back. He immediately came into the room and told me that the lab results were inconclusive but he had some concerns. He wanted to do a lumpectomy to remove the mass. He believed that it would turn out to be malignant. He gave me no reason why other than the swelling under my arm and said that he thought they were related. He proceeded to explain the normal routine of treatment in the event I tested positive for cancer. As he described the latest technology, it seemed as though I was in a tunnel and he was talking to me from outside. My ears picked up only select words such as "chemotherapy" and "radiation". Whatever he said in between was lost in the echoes of those.

My surgery was scheduled for Friday. I was glad. I wanted to get it over with as soon as possible. When I told Dill about my appointment, he asked me if I wanted him to be here with me. I said yes. He started packing.

June 8

I went to the hospital to complete my pre-admission paperwork. While I was there I saw an older gentleman whose face seemed familiar to me. When he sat down in the chair next to mine, he said hello and I recognized his voice, remarkably, as that of my elementary school principal. We chatted and he explained to me how difficult it was to be his age and have back surgery and not be able to play golf and be active enough to enjoy his life. I wondered if he even contemplated the fact that I was there for a medical procedure myself. I wanted to tell him that he should be grateful to live as long as he had. I left the hospital trying to reconstruct memories of what life was like for me in the first grade. I gave up when nothing came to mind.

June 9

Dill arrived early in the morning, tired after driving thirteen hours but smiling and excited to see me. We hugged and when the warmth of his arms surrounded me at that moment I knew for certain that I loved him as something much deeper than a friend. He drove me to the hospital and waited with me in the lobby. Now and then he would glance my way and our eyes would meet. We would gaze at each other for long periods of time and he sent me unspoken messages of love, hope and comfort. The air conditioning was on and I got cold so we moved to sit below a skylight. I rested my head on Dill's shoulder and let the sun shine on my face. I felt at peace.

Even though I come from a large family, not one of my six brothers or sisters was there, nor any of the multitudes of nieces and nephews. My mother was too sick and didn't drive. Jim had threatened if he saw Dill he would punch him. He blamed our marital separation on Dill. Because of that, I told him to stay away. Dill was the one person there for me.

I was soon taken into the pre-op ward and changed into a gown and made to lie on a gurney. My hair was tucked into a blue surgical cap. I was shivering. The nurse spread two heated blankets over me and evaluated my physical and mental condition with a series of questions. She gave me a shot to numb my wrist and then inserted an IV. I thought it odd-giving me a shot to tolerate a needle. Then it was the anesthesiologist's turn and she described the methods she would be using with me. She told the nurse what to give me. The nurse asked her if she had an order. She said, "Yes, it's a verbal one and I just gave it to you." I almost laughed. Her partner came in wearing a brightly colored surgical cap and as he handed the anesthesia to the nurse he smiled and said, "It's Margarita time!". They let Dill come in to see me before wheeling me down to the operating room. I don't remember what was said.

I watched the ceiling tiles approaching like flat clouds and knew I had arrived when just inside the double doors the air around me turned icy. I lifted my head enough I could look around for a brief moment before the medication drug me under. A team of bonneted blue uniforms were pulling on latex gloves and staring at me. The last thing I saw was the cluster of lights above me dancing. If there was any pain I have no memory of it.

What seemed like moments later a stranger was dressing me. She put my socks on crooked and I bent down to straighten them. She walked me to a sitting area where Dill was waiting. The doctor arrived later and without hesitation told me that the surgery went smoothly and the mass had been removed, along with a margin of clean tissue but that his suspicions were accurate. I had cancer. I smiled and said, "Thank you."

As we were leaving, I was given a prescription for hydrocodone, a painkiller. Dill drove me to the pharmacy to get it filled then to the grocery store, then back to my apartment. I sat at the table smoking cigarettes and drinking diet soda while he made pasta salad for us. It was as if I had just been awakened from a confusing dream. I pulled out my address book and began making phone calls. "I had the surgery this morning and it was breast cancer," I repeated time and again. I listened to apologies and stunned silences and was unmoved, unemotional. Afterwards I took my medication and went to sleep.

I had no pain, no discomfort, no nausea, no lightheadedness. The only proof of the surgery was the bandage that wrapped around my breast and under my arm to my back. Over the next few days Dill and I spent countless hours talking, laughing, hugging, and just enjoying being together. One night we went walking on the moonlit beach, holding hands. We found a sailboat and lay side by side on the canvas, looking up at the stars. I confessed to him that I didn't want to die. We both cried.

<u>June 12</u>

I had an appointment to see Dr. Pollard to go over my pathology report but not only was the report not yet available, Dr. Pollard was called away to surgery and so I had to reschedule for the next day.

<u>June 13</u>

Today the nurse removed my bandage to my relief because the itching was annoying me. Dr. Pollard came in and asked me how I was doing. "Great," I said genuinely. I didn't feel like a woman recovering from surgery for breast cancer. I felt like a teenager in love. "How are you?" I asked him, cocking my head and smiling. I wondered if he knew I was sincere. "Been one of those crazy days around here. Your pathology report confirmed Infiltrating Ductal Carcinoma. I will refer you to Dr. Steinberg, an oncologist. He will treat you from here. The plan of attack is to begin chemotherapy with the lymph nodes still intact. If they respond to the chemo, then we remove them. If they don't, we try another type of chemo and hope for better results. That may be all that we need to do, or we may need to go one step further with radiation. Any questions?"

"Yes. How bad is it?" I looked at him. "Why do you want to know that?" he smiled. I laughed incredulously. "Why wouldn't I want to know, wouldn't you?" His face grew serious. "If you are asking me if it can kill you, then the answer is, yes, it could. It is life threatening but that doesn't mean you will die. You have a chance to lead a normal life if the cancer responds to the treatment." I nodded. I had heard nothing that surprised me.

As I approached the front counter to leave, the receptionist stopped me. Her name is Tania. I have known her for a long time. Her eyes were filled with tears. "Betty, I don't know what to say. This is not supposed to happen to women our age." I thanked her and told her I was okay. She told me to go see Dr. Steinberg on Thursday, June 22.

I was happy to get home so that I could finally shower. I had difficulty getting my shirt off because it was stuck to the adhesive still clinging to my skin. I examined my body in the bathroom mirror. My breast was bruised black and blue and covered with yellow iodine. The incision curved around the fullest part and was about four inches long. It was raised and angry and black and pinched tightly closed with perfect clear stitches. I emerged from the bathroom holding a T-shirt to my chest. I found Dill on the balcony reading a newspaper. "Do you want to see it?" I asked him. When he replied, "Sure," I led him into the bedroom and hesitantly moved the shirt aside. "That's not so bad," he said. I walked into the bathroom and dabbed a cotton ball in nail polish remover. I handed it to him and asked if he would be okay helping me clean the adhesive off.

He knelt on the floor beside the bed and told me to sit down. His fingers gently brushed my skin as I watched his face. His eyes were full of love as they moved over me and I felt like my heart would burst. I thought of how Jesus must have felt when Mary anointed his feet in those tender hours before his death. I knew that I was being granted a very rare and special gift in my friendship with Dill. I squeezed my eyes shut and secretly asked God to please let me live.

I thought of my children and how much I loved them and missed being around for them all the time. I knew deep inside that the road I was traveling was going to transform my life and the lives of those around me. Though I didn't know the outcome, I believed that the experience of having cancer would somehow enrich my existence and forever change my focus on the world. I just hoped that I would live to enjoy the aftermath of the process.

June 15

Dill left this morning to go back home. He is out on the road somewhere right now. I wonder what occupies his mind. I wish for him to know how precious he is to me. This past week could have been the saddest, scariest, and most tragic of my life but instead it was full of smiles and happiness. Being around him gave me strength, hope, and courage.

I think about the irony of my situation. When I was healthy and disease-free I was trapped in an unhappy marriage and my only sources of contentment were being with my children and spending money. Now that I have begun to establish some independence and am beginning to embrace love again, I am faced with the raw possibility that I may not be able to continue. I think about tragedy of that and it only makes me more determined to win this. I have more of a reason now to live than I ever have.

I know that I am a strong person. I know that I have the ability to withstand the treatment. I am confident that I have what it takes to pull through this, to fight it, to succeed. I will not allow this disease to take control of my life. As long as I can focus on getting well I believe I will.

June 16

It is 3:41 a.m.

I was in a forest surrounded by darkness. There were figures moving around me but I couldn't see them, only feel their presence. I began darting my eyes, looking around, trying to catch where the movement was coming from. Suddenly I "saw" a ball of invisible energy hurling towards me. I ducked and it missed me but exploded into a tree behind me and the tree burst into flames. I was terrified. I could make out the form of a woman but she was nearly transparent. I knew that she was using psychic powers on me and I realized that if she could, I could too. I summoned all of the strength I could muster and flung my arms out towards her, releasing a wave that knocked her off balance and sent her careening back into the trees. I tried to run but couldn't and then remembered that I could fly. I bolted up off the ground just in time to miss another blast. Then there were several attackers. I rose above the trees; flying low and close enough I could monitor my predators and stay just out of range. I emerged from the woods, barely escaping the assault.

I found myself in a village of dwarflike creatures and they surrounded me, hiding me, protecting me. They moved carefully through the clearing, slowly but steadily, concealing me in their midst, herding their numbers close around me. As we made our way forward, others like them would appear, one at a time, and join us. They were united in trying to get me to safety and did. We reached a big metal door and they opened it for me and I walked through, no longer in danger.

I was standing in a large room where a costume party was being held. It was crowded and people were pushing and shoving their way around me. I recognized faces of girls I went to High School with and thought that I had somehow gone back in time and visited my graduation party. I was looking for some sign of recognition from someone but realized that they could not see me. I was locked in a kind of non-existent plane and couldn't escape. I helplessly stood there as bodies crowded around me and woke up convinced there was someone in my bed, lying close behind me with their body up against mine.

I felt hands on my back, firmly pushing against me. I awakened and tried to move but I was paralyzed. I heard a noise in the kitchen. I tried to lift my head to look and I couldn't. I was gripped with fear. Although I knew it was impossible, I felt the presence of someone. I was not alone. It took all the will I had to finally move a muscle in my leg so that I could turn around. No one was there. The apartment was quiet. After a few moments of silence, I realized that everything was okay but I couldn't shake the feeling of how helpless I was. I wanted to call someone to come over and be with me but realized I had no one I could call. I have never been so alone and afraid as I am at this moment, yet somehow, I know that everything will be okay.

Friday night

Today would have been my first full day back at work since my surgery but because of the nightmares and interrupted sleep last night, I was almost two hours late going in. It was a long day. My arm is giving me pain. I cannot extend it fully and raising it over my head is unbearable. This scares me. I called Dr. Steinberg's office to try and move my appointment up sooner but it wasn't possible.

I am frightened about the near future. I worry about my kids. I know that I will have to give up my full time job. I wonder if I will have to give up my apartment. I have tried to imagine what I would do with my furniture. All these questions and no answers in sight.

What do I tell my children? Do I let them know I am hurting? Should I ease them into the idea that Mommy is sick and may get worse before she gets better? Will she get better? I want to crawl into a deep hole and hide from the world.

I took the kids out to eat Chinese tonight and during dinner my daughter buried her head in my chest and said, "I love you Mommy". I told them both I loved them and said, "How long will Mommy love you?" They answered in unison, "Forever!" Then my son said, "Even if you are gone, like in Heaven, you will still love us." I have taught them that since they were babies. Smart kids. Before we left I cracked open my fortune cookie and read, "An unexpected windfall will be yours". How I want to believe this…

I tried logging on to the Internet to see if Dill was available to chat and was denied access. I called the support tech to see what was going on. I was told that there was a problem with my account. I suddenly thought about bills. I haven't checked my mail in over two weeks now. I just haven't remembered to. I suppose my service has been disconnected for non-payment. I need to pull out of this state of detachment I have found myself in so that I can stay on top of my responsibilities. I do not want to lose any of the pleasures I enjoy now out of sheer neglect. I will do what I can to keep things normal as long as possible.

June 17

I slept last night without dreaming and woke up late. I lay in bed and listened to my children laughing. They are so beautiful. I decided to tell them I was sick. We sat around the kitchen table eating cinnamon toast and talking.

I didn't want to frighten them. They already have fears and sadness about the breakup of my marriage so I wanted to be gentle. I told them that my arm was sore and the doctor is trying to find out why. I explained to them about having my breasts examined and finding a lump and how the doctor decided to cut it out. I said I had surgery and a big ugly scar and asked them if they wanted to see it. They giggled and said yes. When I showed it to them, they made ugly faces and said, "ewwwww gross!"

We laughed about it and I answered as many questions as I could. My son insisted on knowing what it was called but I couldn't tell him. I will eventually talk to them about cancer but right now is too soon. I explained that I would be going to the doctor a lot more and taking medicine that might make me feel bad.

I am relieved to have taken this first step with them.

June 19

My boss Rich has hired a temp worker to "fill in" on the days that I am not there. Of course I am training her to take over for me. Although I have not been fired, nor have I officially quit, there is a silent understanding that Rhoda is replacing me. I am okay with this. I realize that I cannot go through all that lies ahead and still put in the hours I need to in order to do my job. Not only that but I had already decided to look for another job and was in the hiring process at an insurance company for a position with a better salary and benefits.

I am worried about money. I have missed a lot of work because of my doctor visits and surgery. My paychecks are too small now to pay my bills and my rent is due in 11 days. I do not know how I will pay it. I considered moving into my mother's mobile home but that is something I do not want to do. I have worked really hard these past few months to pay my rent and have an apartment of my own. I have sacrificed and done without a lot of things to be self-sufficient and I am saddened by the thought of having to give it all up. I will hold on as long as I can. I have an appointment in ten days to apply for government assistance and disability. In the meantime, I have no idea how I will get by but I am convinced somehow it will work out. Rich advised me to take tomorrow off and try to find a cheaper place to live.

I tried calling Dr. Steinberg's office today to move my appointment up but again they have had no cancellations. This waiting has been hard on me. Every little ache or pain that I experience makes me nervous and scared. Last night after dinner I began having heartburn and then later in the evening, stomach cramps. I took medicine for the heartburn and when it got worse instead of better, I took one of my pain pills. Nothing seemed to help. By midnight I was pacing the floor in tears. I considered going to the emergency room. I guess the medication finally took effect because not long after it was at it's worst it started easing up a little. For a brief moment I wondered if I had been kidding myself thinking I could withstand the rigors of chemotherapy if heartburn and stomach cramps could do this to me. When I woke up this morning though I felt fine and was in a good mood so my spirits were lifted.

June 21

I went to work and pretty much finished up my training with Rhoda. I don't know what else there is to do for me there so I told them to call me if they needed me. I got paid a whopping $73.00 for this week. When I left work I drove straight to the Department of Social Services and put in an application for assistance.

When I left there I went to a helping agency. I asked if there was any type of assistance they could provide for me to help me pay my bills during my treatment. They offered to pay my electric bill, which I happened to have with me. As the woman wrote out the check, she began telling me about her daughter's experience with breast cancer and how she had just had a mastectomy the day before. She showed me a picture of her. I couldn't believe it. This was a girl I had known in High School. The funny thing was, several weeks ago I had a dream and she was in it. I remember waking up wondering why I had dreamt about her. We had not known each other very long and were not really good friends. Another coincidence?

Later I got a call from the human resource director at the insurance headquarters. I have been trying to get a job there and she was calling to tell me they had decided to hire me. I wanted that job so badly! I told her what my situation was and she asked me to call her back when I was through my treatment. I am thankful that this opportunity will be waiting for me when all this is over. It gives me something to work towards.

My breast is irritated and sore, as has been my arm for the past several days. I have worn my bra as instructed constantly since the day of my surgery but it just hurts too badly tonight. I took it off and took a pain pill. Tomorrow is my appointment with Dr. Steinberg. I am hoping that he will give me some kind of clarity about what the future holds.

June 22

This morning I had my first appointment with my cancer specialist.

I have to have a test tomorrow to determine if my heart can withstand the chemo that he wants to use with me. I will be getting a combination of Adriamycin and Cytoxan. Adriamycin is so potent that if it touches your skin it eats through it. Imagine having that pumped into your veins! It is bright red and so the nurses call it the "red devil".

If I pass the test tomorrow I will start my treatments on Monday afternoon. I will be given anti-nausea drugs first, then the chemo. Within the first 24 hours I will start to feel the side effects of nausea, possibly vomiting and diarrhea, and general fatigue. Within 2-3 weeks my hair will start falling out in clumps by the handfuls. I will go once every 3 weeks for 4 rounds. At the end of 12 weeks I will have surgery to remove some lymph nodes and at that point they will be tested. Then I will undergo another 12 weeks of chemo, followed by radiation of the breast. My total treatment time will be about 9 months. Dr. Steinberg warned me that I was in for a "rough ride". I think I am ready.

My visit today cost $733.00. I will apply for Medicaid tomorrow after I go to the hospital. I talked to Jim on the phone when I got home today and told him that I needed more income and that I had no one I could go to for help. He said he would consider what he could do.

I spent most of the night calling people and telling them about my appointment. When I talked to Dill he told me that he was thinking of coming back down. I wonder about what this experience will do to our friendship. I have a hard time accepting the idea that anyone could care about me when I become sick, fat, bald, and on welfare. Aside from that, I think about the risk of investing your heart into a relationship with someone who has a life threatening illness. But when all these thoughts creep into my head, I always come back to the belief that our friendship was meant to be and it is a blessing that I welcome with all my heart.

June 23

This morning I had a test called a muga-scan. This is to determine if my heart muscle can withstand possible damage by chemo. They gave me a shot to make my blood "sticky" then another one a few minutes later to inject a radioactive dye. I had to lie down while the camera moved over me (similar to a CT scan) and images of my heart were taken over a period of about an hour.

I chatted with the technician while she worked. I asked her what her title was. She is a nuclear medicine technologist. She asked if I was considering a career in medicine. I just laughed and said, "well, I don't think so but I do think when this is over I would like to somehow work with cancer patients". She went on to tell me that she did that for several years but had to stop because it was too stressful. She said that it was hard to get close to your patients when you know that 90% of them will die. When I heard this, I decided to ask Dr. Steinberg about those percentages. I want to know statistically what he would say my chances of survival are.

When it was over I asked Luanne if I could see the images. She showed me her monitor and there was my heart, beating strongly. It was incredible. I commented that I wished the image could be printed for me to keep and told her I was writing a diary about my cancer experience. She had never done it before, but it made her curious as to whether or not she could, so we sat down while she tinkered with her printer and managed to print a beautiful full-color glossy copy of the image. She gave it to me and I thanked her and left.

I went to pick up the kids from summer school to take them to visit a friend and on the way my son told me that yesterday he prayed that I would feel better after my doctor's appointment. He is such a sweet loving little guy. I told him that I did feel better after going since I knew now what the doctor was going to do. I said that I wanted to talk to both of them later tonight about it but they wanted me to talk to them right then. I didn't think the car was the ideal place to discuss my chemo but the moment seemed right so I began.

I explained that I had cells in my body that were growing too fast and could cause me to get very sick all over so the doctor had to do something to stop them from growing. He would use a drug that would make me want to throw up and cause my hair to fall out. I promised them I would wear hats and scarves so that they wouldn't be embarrassed about having a bald mommy. They thought this was funny but my son did admit that it scared him a little.

We were stopped behind a truck waiting for the bridge to turn and it just so happened that the man driving the truck was totally bald. I said, "See, that is what I will look like in about 3 weeks." They began naming all the places where I had hair on my body and imagining how I would look totally hairless. My daughter liked the idea of me not having hair on my legs and I told her I liked that idea too. They asked me if it would grow back and I answered that it would but it would take many months. My son said he wished there was something else they could do that wasn't so bad. I agreed with him and said, unfortunately that there wasn't and it was important for me to do everything I could to get well. He calculated that it would be around Christmas before my hair started to grow back and asked if he could stay with his daddy until it did. I almost cried. I just said, "let's see how things go."

<u>June 24</u>

Dill left around midnight to come down here but lost power in his car on the Jersey Turnpike so was delayed for a while trying to get repairs. He made it Saturday evening, very tired. We ordered pizza and just sat around relaxing.

<u>June 25</u>

My sister Bobbi also made it in time for my mother's surgery tomorrow morning and insisted on going with me to my chemo. She has been wonderful and supportive. I love her so much.

June 26

Went to start my chemo today for the first time. Dill and I drove over to the cancer center and Bobbi met us there later. Dill was in the back with me when they got me started on my anti-nausea drugs and when Bobbi arrived he kissed me for good luck. When they started the Adriamycin, I could feel it going into my body like ice. My hand and arm was freezing and I stayed cold for most of the day. Something in the IV gave me double vision and I had a hard time with my coordination for a little while.

June 27

Felt great all day; a little queasy some, but otherwise ok. Today I went out to have some pictures made of myself for the kids before my hair falls out. Dill went with me so we got some pictures made together too. Can't wait to get them!

June 28

Slept through my appointment with Dr. Pollard but had my phone interview with SSA. Looks like I may be able to qualify for some type of disability if my Doctor completes the form appropriately. Also found out I will be getting food stamps in an amount over 300 per month. Things are looking a little better now. And I am hopeful that I will also qualify for Medicaid, which is good since my last visit for chemo cost over 2200!

Today was a little harder than yesterday. I felt tired and a little nauseated but nothing like I imagined I would feel. Dill has been wonderful. He let me rest when I needed to. He brought a puzzle and some videos for us to watch and we had some nice times together. I know that when he leaves town this time it may be a long while before I see him again. I feel that his care and friendship has been vital to keeping my spirits up and when he is gone again I know I will have some rough and lonely days but I also know he has to concentrate on his life for awhile.

He has been so good to me. He is my best friend but so much more. I wish I knew how to thank him. I love him as deeply as I have ever loved anyone. I feel like Dill has been sent to me by God. He is such a blessing. I don't know that I could ever give him what he has given me because I feel he deserves so much. I don't know by what miracle that I am worthy of his love but I try not to question it. I just feel gratitude beyond compare.

<u>June 29</u>

Got a call from Jim today and one of our income tax refund checks arrived in the mail. Thank God for that. I will be able to pay my rent and some of my bills to get me through this month.

Except for some queasiness and being sleepy, I feel pretty good. I am hopeful this will be the rule throughout my treatments. If it does not get worse, and if I do not get financial assistance for some reason, I may feel like taking a part time job. I know it will not be easy but at least I feel like I have some choices now.

Tonight it has rained really hard and I was in the mood to go running on the beach. I put on my windbreaker and shorts and headed out the door. As I was jogging the sun was going down and I marveled at how beautiful the sky was. The thoughts were with me, "This is what life is about. This is what it means to have joy. To run on the beach in the rain and not care about anything else but the steady beat of your heart as it effectively does its job and allows you to see the beauty around you".

<u>July 2</u>

Wow. What a weekend. Where to begin…? Dill has once again gone back home. The last night he was in town we went out to a movie and then to dinner afterwards. We sat in the restaurant overlooking the water. I wanted escargot and he had no desire to eat snails but I fed them to him anyway with his eyes closed. We talked and laughed and I felt good. He was wearing a blue silk shirt and was gorgeous (and of course I told him he was). It was cute because afterwards, we came to the apartment and were sitting on the sofa and he looked at me and asked, "Was that our first date?" It was great to go out and have a good time without thinking about cancer. Especially since later that night I was forced to think about it more than ever since it all started.

That night as I tried to sleep I kept having frightful out-of-body experiences. I woke up several times to run to the bathroom. I was incredibly thirsty...dehydrated. I kept drinking water all night long. The water tasted funny but I thought it was just because I had drunk a glass of wine earlier. In the morning, I had mild stomach cramps. I took my medicine and got on the computer and was chatting with my friend Sal when I suddenly got so sleepy I couldn't continue. I crawled out of my chair and onto the bed, leaving myself online. I don't know how long I slept but the doorbell woke me up.

It was the kids. I let them in and hugged them and then suddenly got hot and dizzy and turned to run to the bathroom. I panicked. Jim tried to come in but I made him wait at the door, not sure if I was going to vomit. I was tired and groggy for the rest of the day and ordered pizza in because I didn't feel like going anywhere. That night I hugged and kissed the kids constantly and ended up sleeping with my daughter in my arms all night.

She was still nuzzled against me when I woke up this morning. As I came out of sleep, I was looking at the watercolor print on my bedroom wall and realized it was unusually fuzzy. I tried to focus and couldn't. I sat up in the bed and let my daughter roll over beside me. I was dizzy. I was nauseated. I was weak. I went into the bathroom to brush my teeth and my gums were sore. The toothpaste tasted bland, not fresh. I went to use the toilet and had diarrhea. I went into the kitchen to take my medicine and couldn't get my water cold enough. No matter how much ice I put in or how much I stirred it, it still felt warm in my mouth. I was scared. I wanted my parents. I wanted to go home.

I called my mother and told her I wanted the kids to celebrate the Fourth of July over there with her and I would bring my laundry to do while I was there. We drove out and bought fireworks and then went to the grocery store and used my food stamps for the first time. I went on to my mom's and made hot dog chili. I couldn't get the taste right. I made Mexican dip with beans and peppers and salsa but it tasted bland. The soda tasted flat. We made ice cream parfaits with vanilla ice cream and red and blue berries but it wasn't sweet enough. Something was wrong with my taste buds.

I spent hours on the front porch with family members while the children played outside. They had a great time and so did I. It was wonderful to be around them. Jim came over and we talked for a long time. He discussed the possibility of my using the divorce settlement money to buy a mobile home and set it up near my mother. I thought about how good it was to have the kids there for the holiday and how scared I had been that morning and realized that I should seriously consider moving.

After the day had ended, I packed up kids, laundry, and food and drove home to the apartment. I poured some lemonade and ate a sugar cookie. I couldn't taste the sweetness of any of it. I sat down at the computer and chatted with Dill. I got up to get ready for bed and realized my legs were swollen terribly. My throat hurts and I have heartburn. I am not looking forward to the rest of the night and tomorrow. I want to sleep but I know I will not. The kids have school tomorrow and I have two doctors' appointments. So far, this has been my worst day because I can feel my body weakening.

July 4

Just got home to a nasty message on my answering machine. Evidently my friend has been trying to call me and was angry with me for not returning her calls. She said some harsh words and I had to stop the tape in tears. I considered dictating her message in this spot so that my reply makes more sense but then I thought better of it for two reasons: I don't want to embarrass her and make her feel worse about it because I care about her feelings and it won't accomplish anything and furthermore I only want to save my reply because it may be helpful in the future for me to remember the feelings I have as a result of what has happened. This was my response to her:

Hey,

I actually just got home after being at my mom's for a few days and have just now listened to your message (by the way, I sent you a message while I knew you were out of town just because I hadn't talked to you in a while and I wanted you to know that I was thinking about you).

I did have company earlier last week. My friend Dill came down for a few days and also my sister Bobbi was here so I was very busy but I returned most of the calls that I received during that time, or at least I tried to. I had so many I was totally blown away and did my best to get to as many as I could. I still have not responded to three or four of the last ones.

I have not ignored anyone, especially you. As a matter of fact, I went out and bought a thank you card for you which is sitting right here on my desk. I haven't mailed it only because I have not been to the post office to buy stamps. I wish I would have done it sooner but I didn't.

I have been touched by your support and concern and I wanted you to know. I have also tried to make it clear to you in the only ways I know how that I do appreciate everything you have done for me.

I hope you realize I cannot just forget that message without talking about it first. I feel like I should be allowed to address some of what you said so here goes:

Please read all of this carefully to the end before you allow yourself to react. First of all, you made an assumption that I was intentionally not calling you without knowing why. Then you got angry with me because you assumed you were right and I had done something wrong. A particularly nasty thing to me was all the harsh words you used on my answering machine for anyone to hear, which fortunately happened to be my children and not some other adult. Even my children were surprised by the things you said. And finally, you made it very clear to me that your "support" was conditional on how I responded. I have to admit this one was the one that hurt me the most. It was as if you were saying in order to earn your concern I would have to act a certain way and that to me is very sad.

I don't know what to say. I love you and I care about you but I am worried too. You are being very controlling to the point that you are willing to hurt people you say you care about. I don't understand this. I was angry at first and I put the tape away because I knew that if I erased it I would one day not remember how horrible it was. But then I thought about it a little more and decided that I don't need to be reminded of it because it would not accomplish anything.

But then I thought I should save it for you because maybe one day you might want to listen to it for your own good. If being a friend to me is causing you this much anguish then please do yourself and me a favor and think about why you are doing it. If you are doing it for me, then you are expecting too much in return. If you are doing it for yourself, then you are not doing it for the right reasons and for that I am truly sorry.

I appreciate every phone call that I get. I have found that people who have not called me in many years are now concerned and calling me. That is wonderful but you also have to realize the reason why. I have cancer. I am not feeling sorry for myself; it's just a fact. No one knows if I am going to live or die and so they are calling. I would too. On my end, my days are long and confusing. I try to be strong and keep up a good front but every moment is a challenge when you don't know what the future holds. Forgive me for not acting in the way that you think I "should".

A lot of people with cancer get depressed. I have thoughts that I know would drive some people crazy. It's no wonder to me that there are people with cancer who commit suicide because I understand how difficult a thing it is to face. But I have faith and I have a healthy outlook on life. I am trying to keep my environment around me as positive as I can right now. That is what I need most. I am not going to try to be selfish and shut people out but if for some reason I did do that, I would hope that in the long run people would somehow understand that if I shut anyone out, it is because they are being detrimental to me. This is not the time in my life when I need unhealthy relationships. If that seems selfish, then perhaps I am selfish. I don't think there is a right way to handle having cancer or a wrong way. I don't think I have ever seen any rules on the subject. Come to think of it, I don't know if there is a right way or a wrong way to be a friend. All I know is I am doing what I have always done and that is to be honest and loving and true to myself and to others. That is me and I don't plan on changing that. I happen to like that about myself very much.

As for our relationship, I do forgive you for the things you said. I understand that you were acting out of your own feelings of frustration. I am sorry for upsetting you and I hope that you are ok now. I have to be honest with you though and tell you that this is probably going to cause me to be more guarded with you, waiting for another attack like that one. It's hard to be fully trusting of someone when they can intentionally hurt you so easily, but I won't shut you out. You have been a lifelong friend and that means too much to me to just let one episode ruin it.

I hope to talk to you soon and this time under more favorable conditions :)

-Betty

I am still reeling by all of the things she said. Emotions are running high around me. I hope that the outcome of this experience is a positive one.

I had my first follow-up appointment with Dr. Steinberg yesterday. They sampled my blood and were pleased with the results. I had a long list of topics I wanted to discuss with him so in my now typical fashion I pulled out my notebook and pen. The side effects from my chemo are more evident now. They are nausea, loose and frequent bowel movements, heartburn, indigestion, dehydration, sore throat (with a reflux type feeling that makes it difficult to swallow and everything I eat seems to get stuck in my throat), loss of taste, sore gums, mouth ulcers, headache, fatigue, and chills. The other symptoms, which are at times just as annoying, are the results of the steroids that are supposed to be lessening the side effects of the chemo. They are swelling, weight gain, cystic acne, interrupted sleep, increased craving for food, dizziness, lack of coordination, and irritability.

I found out that they have officially set me at Stage II, which has about a 78% ten year survival rate. They are not simply treating me but are attempting a cure. The surgery under my arm will be done to remove lymph nodes for testing, but also to remove the obvious cancer there. This was new information for me. Up until now I had not been told that the swelling was indeed cancer. He referred to it as a secondary tumor. When I questioned this, he explained that the "mother" tumor was the one in the breast that had been removed and this cancer was the offspring. Although it is not necessarily one "tumor", it is a cancerous mass that is a conglomeration of lymph nodes and possibly other involved tissue.

He did tell me that other than the inevitable impending hair loss, I have felt the severity of whatever side effects I will have throughout my treatment. This was encouraging to me. He told me that I was doing great and he was proud of me and I consider it to have been a good visit.

When I left the office I went by the apartment to pick up some things before going to get the kids and ran into my landlord. I discussed with him the idea I had about possibly buying a mobile home in the near future. He told me that if he was able to find a tenant to take over the apartment then I would no longer be obligated to my lease and that he actually did have someone who wanted to move in the beginning of August. The longer I wait beyond then the less my chances will be of getting someone because of the fact that summer will be winding down and there will be fewer renters in the market then.

With this in mind, I went back to my mom's and discussed with her more seriously the idea of moving out there. We decided that if things were to go in that direction, I would most likely have to put my furniture in storage temporarily and move in with her until I could get a mobile home set up. The big question is will I be able to get my settlement money from Jim in time? I called him and talked to him about it. He agreed to go to the bank this week and find out what he can do. He will most likely have to take out an equity loan on the house.

I had a conversation with Dill about this because I trust his opinion and asked him to share his concerns with me, which he did. The two negative aspects he could offer were:

1) Not wanting me to feel that I had once again been forced to go to Jim as my "savior" and thus feeling some further dependence, obligation, or emotional attachment to him and
2) Not wanting me to be placed in an environment around members of my family that could be emotionally draining to me and compromise the positive surroundings I have been so adamant about having during my treatment.

I was thankful for his input because it did make me think about my priorities and help me get some perspective on them. Although his concerns are legitimate, I think under the circumstances the advantages far outweigh the disadvantages. Not only that, but I imagined the details of setting up a house there and got really excited about it. I considered what it could do for my spirits to be situated in a permanent place of my own where I would not have to be concerned about rent or moving again at the beginning of the year. I thought about celebrating Christmas in a new place with my children and family around me and the image was intensely rewarding. In addition to all that, I think the experience of beginning a new year at the end of cancer treatment in a new home with a new job nearby is something I could greatly look forward to.

I ended up cooking dinner at my mom's and talking long into the night with her. I had to go to the store and when I got back the children were asleep so we spent the night over there. I slept well and woke up thinking that I was certain I was making the right decision.

July 6

Woke up again this morning with an intense headache. Ate breakfast with the kids and got them off to school. I went by the beauty salon where my sister in law gets her hair done. The owner of the salon has received community service awards for her charity work with the American Cancer Society and she is having a benefit golf tournament this weekend to raise money. She works closely with breast cancer/chemo patients in the Look Good Feel Good program where her staff helps choose and style wigs and teach women like me how to cope with the physical challenges of chemo, offering beauty tips and training on how to wear scarves and turbans, etc. I met Lou and she pulled out a wig that she had in the back that she was willing to give me. It was dark brown; the same color as my natural hair and was long and braided in a French braid down the back. On the form, it was like I was looking at the back of my head. It made me feel good. I have an appointment with her on Tuesday afternoon for her to fit it on me and trim it and show me how to fix it. I hope my hair holds out until then. It is beginning to come out now. When I run my fingers through it, several strands come out between my fingers and I am noticing loose hairs on my shoulders more.

This afternoon I had to go to the Cancer Center to have my blood tested and my white blood cell count was dangerously low. They gave me a shot to hopefully stimulate my bone marrow production. The shot was a painful one and they said I would experience discomfort by tonight and pain in my bones as my body began responding. I have to go back in tomorrow, Saturday, and maybe Sunday for more injections like that one and to have my blood tested again. They also put me on strong antibiotics because of my high risk of infection right now. When I went to check out, the bill for the shot was two thousand dollars. I thought it was a misprint. I showed it to the girl. It was right. And I have to have three more this week.

After I left there, I went to Dr. Pollard's office. When he came into the room he asked me, "So what's the word?" I just shook my head and said, "Can't think of one to use that covers everything," He laughed and said, "I've got one for ya. S-H-I-T. Shit." I laughed and said, "Yup, that one will work just fine." He examined my incision and said it looked good. The stitches are almost dissolved and no further care is needed for my surgery. He said he would see me at the end of my chemo to schedule the surgery on my underarm. Before I left I passed out crispy rice treats to Tania and the other girls in the office.

My mother took me out to dinner and I ate a steak. We sat around the restaurant drinking coffee and talking. These times have been good for us. We have managed to get along well and enjoy one another's company. I am thankful for this.

We went back to her house and I had a message from the woman who owns the land for rent out there. She lives across the street from my mother and walked over. We talked about the lot I liked and she gave me an application to fill out if I wanted to lease it. She said she would hold it for me for a couple of weeks without a deposit and give me time to decide what I am going to do.

I came home and called Jim to tell him that I am in for a rough weekend and need him to go ahead and pick up the kids as scheduled tomorrow afternoon. He had asked me to keep them because he wanted to go out of town but I thought that in light of the day I had today he would be willing to postpone his trip or at least make other arrangements for them. He wasn't willing to do that and I was angry. I told him I would watch the kids but I left him with some choice words and then hung up on him. I hate doing that. I feel badly about allowing myself to get angry but more than that, I regret not standing up for myself and resentfully agreeing to do it anyway even though I know it is not a good idea. I just wish I could have more clarity when I talk to him. Every conversation with him is a reminder of how poor the communication was in our marriage.

I have thought a lot about the impact all this is having on Jim and I know that he is going through a difficult time. I feel badly for him. His mother died from cancer when he was 14 years old and I am sure he is terrified. He is keeping his feelings deep inside and this worries me. The past several months have been really hard on him. He is concerned about me and I know in his heart he wants to help me somehow but he is also dealing with the hurt and anger of my leaving him. He feels like he wants to be there for me but by doing so he is making himself vulnerable because I think he still cares and it only causes him further heartache. It is too soon into our separation for him to feel like he can be a friend to me without expecting me to be his wife in return and I understand this.

I wish things were simpler. Although I do care about him, I get frustrated with him very easily. I am trying to be more patient and understanding with him but it is hard. In his mind, he is bending over backwards to help me although he thinks I am acting ungrateful. In fairness to him, I have to say that he is dealing with things the best way he knows how and I can see how he feels he is making an effort.

I feel sad that our marriage is over. I abhor divorce and what it does to a family. I don't like the idea of my children having their lives torn apart. I never imagined I would be in this situation. I wanted so badly to make it work and I believed for many years that it could. I look back now and can see that I was in denial about how unhappy I was.

At one time we had a lot of dreams and ambitions. Having our children was an incredibly rewarding experience and Jim proved to be a wonderful father. He is hardworking. He gets along well with people. He started out with no experience or education in his field and became a good businessman. I was intensely proud and supportive of his accomplishments. He accomplished a lot during our marriage. For 13 years I was willing to be content with the life that we had. But I realize that as time went by and I got older I began to want more from my marriage emotionally.

We took one another for granted. We were too comfortable. Jim and I were more like casual friends than husband and wife and although I believe friendship is the foundation for a good marriage, I also believe it has to go far beyond that. We started out as "partying buddies" and there was a lot of drug usage involved. We were more desperate for companionship than attracted to one another. I felt like we never had a real spiritual connection. I never felt like he understood me or wanted to. We never just sat down and talked to each other. I never felt like we were "in love". I felt unappreciated. It was as if I was a bystander in my own life, waiting for something to happen to make me feel like my life had finally begun. I never felt like the affection, passion, and devotion I showed him was being returned. After living with that for so long, I began to feel the void and resent him for it.

By the time it became apparent to him that our relationship was in trouble, I was already too far detached emotionally to be willing to make the effort to try and save it. We did go to marriage counseling for a brief time but even that was difficult because of how poorly we communicated.

The therapist would ask me a question about my feelings and Jim would answer. It was as if I wasn't capable of speaking my own mind. He said he knew me better than I knew myself. I tried it a couple of times and finally threw up my hands. I refused to go back to the marriage counselor. I know that he will always blame me for this and feel like I didn't give him the opportunity to change things before I gave up on it.

I hope that my children will one day understand that I had to leave the relationship in order to find myself and grow personally outside of his control. I have never wanted to cause heartache. I have always tried to avoid that. I believe that love is the most important thing in the world and it hurts me to know that my actions have caused pain to others. I am sorry for making Jim and the kids sad but I had just reached a point where I felt like I was dying inside (which in actuality I was).

Since I left Jim I have renewed some of my old friendships and this has given me a lot of pleasure. People that I know have been supportive and kind to me. My friends have shown a great deal of concern for me. I get letters and cards and packages in the mail. I have received books from some people and one of them talks about the possible connection between living a toxic emotional life and having cancer. It gives examples of women just like me who, after years of surviving in stressful and unhealthy relationships end up with cancer during the separation period. It's interesting to consider the correlation that may exist there.

I merely existed in circumstances that were unhealthy and unsatisfying. It is my hope that this experience will change all that and I can look forward to living a healthier and happier life all the way around.

<u>July 7</u>

I had a restless night last night and couldn't sleep. I thought about having the kids this weekend and how weak and tired I feel and I knew I needed to insist that Jim keep them. I called him at 7 this morning. He told me I "had to" pick up the kids from school so he could go out of town and I said, "no I DON'T have to and I am NOT". Although I did not want to do this, I felt it was the only choice I had. He was angry of course and accused me of simply being inconvenienced by having to pick them up and intentionally trying to ruin his trip out of jealously (I didn't realize he was going out of town with another woman). I couldn't believe this. I think I am handling this illness extremely well so far and I am disappointed that he can't just understand that I don't feel well enough to do it this time.

July 8 (morning)

Another restless night last night. I have to say last night was the worst so far. When I went to the cancer center for my appointment yesterday they took my temperature and it was 101. They are very concerned about this and told me to go back home and lie down and not go anyplace where I would be around people. They cautioned me not to let anyone come visit me either, especially children and told me it would be best if I just stayed inside all weekend. It appears I made the right decision to not be around my kids.

I was instructed to take my temperature often and monitor it. If it goes up any, I am to call them immediately. When I got home I realized I didn't have a thermometer and mentioned this to my niece when I talked to her on the phone later. She showed up at my apartment, rang the doorbell and left me a bag with magazines and a thermometer. I was touched by this. She has been very sweet lately.

Before I went to bed, I ran my hands through my hair out of habit and when I saw how much hair stuck between my fingers it sent me into tears. I began tugging at individual strands and they just let go with very little resistance. I know that if I grabbed a section and pulled on it, it would come out. I wonder how much worse it will be by Sunday. I really wanted to see the kids again before it came out and I wish there was some way I could take them with me to get it cut so it will be less of a shock to them but I can hardly move around, much less get so ambitious as to do that. Besides, I am not supposed to have contact with people anyway.

Although I have been expecting this and have tried not to let it get me down, I couldn't help getting upset about it. Even though at times I have been unhappy with my body and my looks I have always loved my hair. People have always complimented me on how beautiful my hair is and now I am facing losing the one thing I could count on when nothing else about my appearance was good enough for me.

As the night progressed, I became achy and restless and sometime in the night the pain in my back, hips and jaw got so severe it woke me up. I tossed and turned and had fitful dreams. This morning when I got out of bed I took my temperature and it was just under 100. I cannot get into a comfortable position where I do not hurt somewhere. Lying down is the worst and sitting up isn't much better.

I have an appointment at 11:00 this morning to go back and get my last shot and have my blood tested. For the first time since I got sick I am not sure how I will manage getting dressed, maneuvering the staircase, and driving myself over there. It is clear to me today that I need to be closer in proximity to my family for the days like this when I physically need someone to help me.

<u>July 8 (evening)</u>

Well my appointment did not go exactly as I hoped it would. The acceptable range for a platelet count is between 130 and 400 (thousand I think) and my platelet count was 118. This means I will have to have more shots. I got one today and have to go back tomorrow, Monday and probably Tuesday. The nurse told me that she hated to be the one to break it to me but that this would probably be a pattern for me following each chemo treatment. Five days of that damned injection each time and the accompanying fevers and seclusion. I am irritated. I feel my determination to beat this being undermined by my body's lack of cooperation.

I know I need to do something more but I don't know what. Surely there is a supplement I can take or a diet I can adhere to that will boost my immune system. I know I need to quit smoking and I am trying. I know I need to meditate and practice imagery. I feel like I should be exercising, walking or something. This is so frustrating. Yes, I am going to do everything I can to win this but damnit once in awhile I just want to get mad about it. I will let myself feel these feelings without punishing myself for them.

July 11

I am doing much better today. I went and had my shots over the weekend and yesterday my platelet count was 181 so I didn't have to have another shot and I cancelled my appointment for today. This will be a 6-day stretch of no doctor appointments and no needles! Yay!

This morning I had to go to the attorney's office to amend my separation agreement with Jim to allow the early distribution of our marital assets. I came home and took a nap and then got up in time to go to my hair appointment.

Lou cut all my hair off so that it is about an inch long all over. She had a hard time doing this. She said my hair was beautiful and she just hated to be the one to cut it all off. I tried to make her feel comfortable and encouraged her to keep cutting, shorter, shorter still. The hair on the floor was unbelievable! She fitted me with a wig. It was bulky and old fashioned looking but I came home and pulled out my scissors and started whacking on it. The bangs don't hang quite right and Sue scorched them when she tried to curl them with the curling iron but I managed to cut most of that out. It actually looks very much like my hair now and it will be sufficient. At least I no longer have to worry about being bald around the kids and that is a big relief.

I can hardly believe I have almost a week of no treatments or injections and I am not quite sure what to do with myself!

July 15

I have had a good week in terms of how I was feeling physically but emotionally it was a struggle. My hair is coming out in tufts by the hundreds. There is hair everywhere in my apartment. My shoulders stay covered with it no matter how often I brush it away. It is all over my bed, all around the floor by my computer…I stand in the bathroom to brush my teeth and before I leave I have to wipe out the sink. I just stand there and watch it collect. I have bald spots all over my head.

When I got home with the wig I felt better about having it but it was a different story when it came to actually wearing it. I kept myself inside for two days and didn't go anywhere because I was so self-conscious. I realized what was happening and one night I put on a bandana and made myself go take out the trash and then drive to the store.

Yesterday I got up and took a shower and put on my makeup and my wig. I was headed out the door and noticed my landlord's door open so I went over to say hello. When I walked in, he said, "I see you got your new hair." Because he hasn't seen my hair since it started coming out, it meant that the wig was obvious and was a little disappointing. I just laughed it off and changed the subject. I told him that I was most likely going to try and move September 1st and would confirm that with him within the next couple of weeks.

Then I went to pick up the kids from school and was very much aware when I was talking with the teacher that she was trying not to look at me and was unusually talkative. The kids were happy to see me and when we got into the car they said that their daddy had told them my hair was short now and so they didn't expect to see me with long hair. I told them it was a wig and it made me feel good that they hadn't realized it wasn't my own hair. We went over to my mom's and she said that it looked like my natural hair (but of course she cannot see very well, so it was not that encouraging!). We went out to dinner together and it was a little uncomfortable for me. Most people of course didn't notice but some stared just a little too long. I'm not sure that I wouldn't just rather wear a baseball cap.

Last night the kids had a light-hearted curiosity about my hair and I was glad that they were not overly concerned about it. I took the wig off just a little so they could see my balding scalp and then I let them take it off the rest of the way. Scarlett wanted to wear the wig so I let her. They both wanted to pull some of my hair out so I let them. Scarlett told me I was still pretty and that she could tell I was her mommy because of my eyes and my smile. I was really happy they took it so well.

<u>July 19</u>

Monday I took the kids into school and was running late so just plopped on a baseball cap. They were fine with that…I have been "bareheaded" with them since I picked them up so that they are used to the way I look. I did notice a few stares from other parents at school but just shrugged them off.

My sister Bobbi drove up from Georgia to be with me for a couple of days this week. She took me to chemo on Monday morning. The nurses were stunned to see how fast my hair had fallen out but of course were very sweet and encouraging, telling me I looked "cute" in a cap.

Dr. Steinberg examined me and said he felt like my lymph nodes were shrinking! Thank You God! I had a good visit and the "Red Devil" Adriamycin didn't effect me as much as it did the last time. I guess a lot of the fear has lessened.

After chemo, we went to a sandwich shop and I ate lunch. I think this was a good idea…I didn't feel quite as queasy as last time. We then went to get my prescriptions from the pharmacy and then I came home and rested before going to my hearing with Jim.

He came to pick me up and I was wearing a dress and a hat. He was in a good mood and we drove to the courthouse cordially, although I didn't say much. His driving was making me nauseated and at one point he had to slam on his brakes to keep from hitting the car in front of us, which caused a wreck immediately behind us.

We got into the courtroom and the judge was a young woman. She went over the separation agreement and when she reviewed our financial statements she became concerned. She asked me if I thought it was fair and I answered, "yes ma'am". She asked about my illness. She told me that I should be asking for alimony and more child support and she ended up throwing the document out of court and closed the hearing, shaking her head. She apologized for the inconvenience. Jim was furious. He shoved his chair really hard into the table and slammed the door as he was leaving. Both the judge and the Bailiff looked at me with compassion in their eyes and said good luck to me as I left.

On the way back home, Jim spoke very little. He was angry. He had been telling me that because I was the one who left, he didn't owe me a dime. I felt like I had been avenged. I asked for very little, accepted all his concessions, went into it honestly, didn't ask for any more, and came out feeling like I was being honored for it. I don't know what will happen from here but if today was a gauge then I feel like I am on the right track.

Of course I am worried that Jim will try to use my friendship with Dill to avoid paying me alimony and possibly even contesting my child custody rights. Although he has nothing that he could use to prove my relationship with Dill is anything other than friendship, I still have concerns. With enough money and a good attorney there is more injustice than justice in the law.

As a result of this encounter today, I had a talk with Dill. Even though he wants to move down here to be closer to me during this illness, I don't think it is a good idea now. It is so sad. I want to be nearer to him. He has been so good for me. But I know that I will have to get by without his companionship. This may be the longest six months coming up that I have ever had to face in my entire life. I just hope that I can be strong and withstand all the weak and lonely moments I am bound to feel.

Speaking of weak moments, while Bobbi was here we tried to cram a lot of activity into two days. Although we didn't do all that much, it was tiresome for me. We went out to breakfast and I noticed the manager staring at me. I thought I recognized him. When we went to check out, I saw his business card and realized I went to high school with him. I chatted a bit but could tell he was uncomfortable.

Later that day Bobbi and I went to see a movie together for the first time in over 20 years and both had fun. While we were there, the concession stand worker had a hard time looking at me. At one point Bobbi went to the restroom and I found myself alone in the lobby. I couldn't help but feel self-conscious as the eyes roamed to me then over me then away.

When we stopped at the grocery store on the way home, I was standing at the checkout with just a few items and the woman behind me kept her grocery cart loaded until I began walking away. Even the cashier seemed to drop the change into my hand as if she didn't want to touch me. I feel like people think I am a freak. I mentioned this to Bobbi and she said, "They probably think you have AIDS." I can understand.

We ended up at my mom's one night and Bobbi cooked dinner for all of us. My son had decided to stay with his dad so it ended up being just the girls…me and Bobbi, and my mom and my little girl. She had a great time helping Bobbi batter fried chicken and it was really sweet. I lay down on the sofa while they worked and felt good that I was making the effort to be closer to my family.

Last night the kids were rowdy and I couldn't get them settled down. They stayed up way too late. Making dinner for them was exhausting and I wanted to go to sleep. This morning I stayed in bed until noon and let them eat cereal on their own. I finally got up and cooked a nice lunch but knew I had a long day ahead. Jim called to see how I was doing and I asked him if he would consider letting them spend the night with him for a couple of days. He was agreeable with this. I was so thankful. When he got here around 5pm I was lying down on the sofa and still in my nightgown. Hopefully he will be more understanding and patient with me. I just cannot go full swing all the time anymore.

July 20

When I first discovered the swelling under my arm I had no doubt it was cancer. Although I was frightened, I did what I normally do and I thought through it logically. Instead of asking God, "why me?" I found myself asking God "why NOT me?". I have always been stubborn. I have always been determined. Somehow, no matter what life hands me, I have always had this unshakable faith that something good would come from it and I would bounce back. I know that I am the very type of person who could not only handle this disease, but benefit from it as well.

I grew up poor. I know what it is like to go from day to day not knowing what hardship tomorrow will bring. There was little material or emotional comfort in my young life. My father was an alcoholic and my mother was always sick. Yet, it seemed, with my father's unshakable faith in God and constant prayer, things always worked out. We never had an abundance of anything but it seemed we always got what we needed to get by at the time.

As I grew up and away from that influence of my parents, I began to lose some of that inner trust in God. I began to become impatient and want more from the world. I turned my back on my upbringing and somehow thought I was meant for better things. At times I was ashamed of my past and wanted desperately to run from it. I always hoped that one day I would break away from the "bondage" that poverty had imparted on me and live a deeply gratifying life.

My marriage seemed to offer me all that I wanted. My husband had a good job and we had two beautiful kids, the house with the white picket fence, the family dog and cat, the nice sedan and an SUV, money to spend, and a bright future. But I wasn't happy. I had accomplished nothing. My personal ambitions were still waiting to be tested. I would spend hours just thinking about all the things that I knew I was capable of that I was not doing because I was too comfortable with my life. I was afraid to act because I was afraid to make waves and threaten the "good thing" I had finally found.

A few months ago when I was newly separated from Jim, I spent a lot of time in deep thought about my faith. In the last months of my marriage I had begun questioning the very existence of God. I was raised to believe in God and I was taught to pray and find comfort in Him. I had not done this in many years.

I knew that my life was in trouble. I knew that something had to change. I felt like I was a bird in a cage, dying for freedom. All I knew to do was get out, get away from my circumstances and try to see my life from a perspective that was not clouded by my husband's opinions of what was right and wrong for me. I had let him dominate my thinking for so long. I had gotten to the point where I felt I could no longer even make decisions on my own.

One night in desperation I went to God in prayer. I told him that I was sorry I had shut him out of my life and that I wanted very badly to have faith. I asked him to help me. I asked him to give my life some direction. I always felt I was capable of more than I had become and I asked him to help me discover the gifts he had given me. I asked him to teach me patience. I asked him to help me find some peace and joy in the little things in my life. I asked him to help me finally experience what life was all about. That is about the time I found the lump under my arm.

I realize that this experience of having cancer could actually be turned into something positive. I do not believe God waves his hand and inflicts disease upon us but I do believe that if having something like this can help accomplish His will he may allow it to happen. I am definitely learning patience. I have begun to embrace small joys as they come. Life is much more precious to me.

I know now that I could work with people who have life threatening illnesses. I believe that there is a professional calling in this for me somehow. I know I have a gift for being a friend, a confidant, a listening ear. This is evident in all my friendships and has been most of my life.

When I started college I majored in psychology. I wanted to be a counselor but ended up changing my major to education because I didn't know if I could make it to graduate school in order to be a licensed therapist. I knew I could work with people, teaching them. I did keep social studies as my focus because of my interest in psychology, but when I did not get a teaching job after graduation I simply gave up on the idea. I began to question why I had chosen education in the first place. Going through college was exciting and made me proud but in the end left a void in my life.

Another unfulfilled dream of mine is to be a published author. I always did well in English and Literature and discovered that I did have a knack for writing. For many years I have longed to write but had no idea what to write about. I often thought, "If only I had experienced something that would give me a good subject for a book". I never imagined I would be going through what I am now but one thing I realize is that I DO have a topic now that others may be interested in.

This illness is giving me a new direction. I realize how important it is to have dreams and ambitions. I don't think about a future filled with sickness. I think about a future filled with hope. I want to make the most out of my life.

July 24

Spent all weekend over at my mom's. I was just so tired. Jim came over on Saturday and got the kids early. I stayed in bed most of the day but by yesterday I was restless.

I ended up doing a lot of cleaning, cooking, and laundry and realized that I needed to come home to the apartment and use some of that energy around here!

I went to the cancer center today and got my CBC (complete blood count) and everything was good. I stopped by the pharmacy on the way home. I bought some survival essentials: lip balm, vitamins, soup, yarn, and a funny movie.

It has been storming off and on since Friday night. I have had trouble regulating my body temperature. My head gets cold at night and I find myself burrowing under the covers to keep warm. I have had a runny nose since Saturday and am doing everything I can to not get sick this week. I am taking Beta Carotene, Vitamin C, Co-Enzyme 10, Vitamin E, Melatonin, B-12, and a Multi-Vitamin. I am also drinking a powdered vitamin drink.

July 28

Day 11 after my chemo my white blood count dropped to .4 with 2.0 being the lowest acceptable. I am facing another weekend of shots, fevers, antibiotics and isolation but I am not concerned with those. What occupies my mind is my divorce.

Two nights ago Jim called and threatened me. He was angry and screaming at me over the phone. He warned me that if I did not sign an agreement relinquishing my rights to alimony that he would haul me into court for litigation and sue me for adultery. I was stunned. Although he has no proof of this, he believes that he can substantiate an "emotional affair of the heart" as a basis. He believes that I will get absolutely nothing and he will get custody of the children. Evidently a member of his family saw me walking with Dill when he was here in a public place holding hands and they told him.

People are telling me not to worry, that he cannot possibly succeed but I am concerned. He has hired the best attorney in town. I have asked friends and relatives for recommendations on attorneys and no one has any confidence that a local attorney can win against him. My best chance to fight him is a lawyer who practices in the state capitol, 2 ½ hours away. I found her telephone number and made an appointment for Wednesday. I do not want to fight but I'll be damned if anyone will use my children to try and blackmail me.

August 2

Tomorrow is my appointment with the attorney. Tonight I wrote out a list of questions I have, trying to get prepared. I have thought about nothing else for the past several days except that my actions following this meeting will set the tone for my future dealings with Jim. I realize that my whole future is riding on how I choose to deal with this separation. It is an awesome responsibility; one that I wish I did not bear.

Before I went to bed I prayed. I asked God to give me clarity and good judgment. I asked him to be with the attorney as she was advising me and to help me make a decision that would be in the best interest of the children.

3:13 a.m.

I wake up and I am in my bed in my former home. My children are in the bed with me. A stranger comes into the room and we pretend to be asleep. He is uniformed and armed and we are afraid even though his actions do not seem threatening. He checks to see that we are sleeping and then exits the room. When we are sure that he is gone, we climb up to the window to peek out and see if we can see him outside.

We see his commanding officer sitting outside on a bench where he can monitor our actions outside the window. The yard is fenced in and we are sure that there are guards at the doors and the gate. I see myself walk outside to talk to the officer. I realize than that I am two people. I am both my mother and myself; the parent and the child, and I am frightened. My parent self is going to try and negotiate with these strangers, putting on her most sincere and humble front. She is offering them tea and coffee and hospitality and while she is talking I am watching her from the window.

I can feel her apprehension and her anger. I know what she is doing is risky. She is putting herself in great danger to try and negotiate with them but I know she is doing it to protect all of us. She is biding time, trying to show them that she has no intention of being a threat to them. She is trying to keep a peaceful atmosphere because she knows that if anyone opposes them they have the power to destroy us and she is afraid of them taking the children. She is determined to bring us through this peacefully.

She comes back inside and sits on the bed with me, comforting me, quieting me. She tells me that it is the only way and that I must go along with her plan. She pleads with me to stay where I am and be patient and quiet. She hugs me and rocks me and promises that things will get better soon if I do as she says.

I got out of bed dumbfounded. I prayed for an answer and then I had this dream. What I feel in my heart I must do has never been clearer than at this moment. I have to keep my anger under control. The welfare of the children is the most important factor in my divorce. Whatever decision I make has to remain centered around that priority.

<u>August 23</u>

Since my last journal entry my life has been like a whirlwind.

I did go see my attorney in out of town. I explained to her that I simply wanted what was fair and just in the eyes of the law and we worked out some amendments to the separation agreement that we felt Jim would hopefully agree to. It turns out she is good friends with his attorney and was actually going to see him while on vacation the following week and said she would take my file with her and discuss it with him.

As it turns out, Jim was not able to get the entire amount of my settlement with his loan. Not only that, but he is not willing to release the money until our agreement is final. As much as I wish I could go ahead and move, it looks like that will not be possible for some time to come.

I have accepted that I am just going to have to be patient and see what works out. In the meantime, I have been busy trying to have good quality time with the kids when they are with me and in the other times simply getting enough rest.

My last chemo was uneventful. Of course it is always uncomfortable, especially when the Adriamycin hits my veins. I get so cold then. Bobbi was with me again and we went out to lunch afterwards. She was nauseated and not feeling well so I took her home early. We had some discussion about how my illness has drawn us closer. She has been more like a sister to me lately than ever before in my life.

I have spent a lot of time over the years wishing my family life was different. Out of 7 half-brothers and sisters I feel that Bobbi is the only one I can depend on. Most of the others I have very little contact with, even though most of them live in my same town. One has died. One half-brother lives next door to my mother and even though I see him quite often, we never talk or do anything together. Although he asks my mother about how I am doing regularly, he does not call me since he found out I have cancer. Neither does another of my half-sisters that at one time I felt I was very close to.

I have tried over the years to get closer to her but it seems like it is always me making the effort and my efforts are never returned. She recently began sending me emails, asking how I was doing but they are not even personalized with a greeting. I have always thought of her as a cold, unfeeling person and her emails reflect that. After getting several of these from her, I began to get angry.

One night in particular, I was heavily medicated because of the pain in my bones and I responded with a painfully honest and hurtful email. These are the emails:

Her-*Please let me know how you are doing!!! I'm concerned about your physical and emotional state.*

Me-*How am I doing? Hmmm....Well, right now I am feeling like I have a hangover. I haven't slept in a few days so Doc. gave me sleeping pills....they work really well cause I didn't get out of bed today until 6 pm.*

My emotional state??? Sometimes I laugh, sometimes I cry. I am strong, I am open-minded, and I am determined. If anybody can get through this, I know I can. There are things that I wish were different that I cannot change. But I am dealing with things the best way I know how.

You know, there are a lot of things I don't understand. Like why, for example, you express concern for me and say you have tried to call yet I have been separated from my husband for 8 months and have not received one call from you yet HE has received calls from you (I know this because I was at the house one day when you called him to ask how he was doing). At the birthday party, why did you go up and hug him in front of everyone and not even say hello to me???

Why, when I accepted an invitation from my mother for me and my daughter (your niece) to go and have dinner at her house that day our Aunt was down, did I do something so terribly wrong that it caused you to be furious? Did you not consider that my kids and I have no money and a meal with my family was something that I was grateful for? I didn't know you had paid for that food but even so; if my children were hungry would you not offer them food?

Why, when I needed to borrow money from my mother to help pay my bills did you all but refuse to help? Would you not do the same for your daughter? Are you not the least bit understanding about the fact that I am experiencing some desperate times financially? Do you blame me for leaving my husband? Why does your opinion about my marriage allow you to judge me?

Do you not recall the years that I shared my bed with your daughter so you could have a place to live and work and someone to watch her so you could work and go out at night? Do you think that was easy for me? For all of us? But yet we did it because we loved you and her and you needed us. Where is that gratitude?

I tried recently to reach out to you about my cancer. I was scared because my hair was falling out by the handfuls. I called a few people in my family because I wanted to visit them. Your excuse to not let me come over was WHAT??? Give me a break. Could you not have explained that your sister had cancer and wanted to see you for a few minutes? That was the final blow, the lowest insult.

I see your emails expressing concern but I have difficulty swallowing it. Where has your concern been for me my entire life??? I am sorry but I can't help but feel you are acting out of either obligation or guilt. You've never loved me and you have made it obvious. So obvious, in fact, that I should have given up a long, long time ago but I didn't.

I have tried to reach out to you and overlook little things that happen and continue to love you over the years and every time I do I get my hand slapped. I am tired of playing your little games. My life means too much to me now to allow you to continue to hurt me.

If you really wanted to know how I was doing you would have made the effort to find out long before now. Thank you for finally coming around but it's only a matter of time before I do something else to piss you off and then I will be on your shitlist again. No thank you.

Sorry, but I've been this route with you too many times. Thanks for your concern but it is not necessary.

Her response back?

You are not the only one tired of trying to have a relationship that never seems to work out. Guess you and I are just too different.

Good luck and Good bye.

There is a lot in there that needs explaining. Evidently she has had quite a lot of communication with Jim and members of his family because she knows details about our separation and such that she could not find out anywhere else. Additionally, he had spread a rumor that I was having an affair and that is why I left. It was totally untrue but I think a lot of people believed him. This makes me feel betrayed that she can call and talk to him but not even call me.

Her anger over my having dinner with my mother was because she had arranged the dinner and had not invited me but my mother did, not realizing it would make her mad. When she got there and saw me, she left without explanation because she was furious that my mother invited me without her permission.

In regards to the money situation, my mother has a savings account in her name. She cannot make a withdrawal without her signature. When my mom agreed to loan me money, she had a fit and refused to get the money until after arguing with my mother and several days of waiting, she finally gave in.

One day I asked her if I could come by and visit because I wanted to see her before I was bald and she said her married boyfriend was over and had been given a Viagra pill by a friend and they wanted to test it out and so I could not come over!

The bottom line with her is that she has made no effort through the years to be neither friend nor sister to me and not only that, but has been outright hurtful by her actions. I got to the point where I decided I had put up with it for long enough without at least voicing my feelings. Well, true to form, instead of addressing my questions to her and considering the fact that I am in a highly emotional state, she got extremely angry and told my mother and other members of the family that I had disowned her.

Although I feel badly about the result, I cannot say I regret what I did. I have dealt with feelings of rejection from her my entire life. If I don't do anything else as a result of having cancer, I will try to emotionally detach myself from the people in my life who cause me pain. I wish the outcome could have been one of communication and problem solving but in this case I suppose it just can't happen. It is no wonder to me that she has lived alone for so long. I really can't think of anyone that could put up with her nasty attitude. I have had to reassure myself time and again that I have done the right thing. I hope that one day maybe she will understand but I think that is too much to hope for. Since all this happened I have just prayed that God will somehow work it out.

August 24

When I began considering counseling as a career option recently, I found out that I would have to go to graduate school to get a master's degree. I knew my chances were slim because not only do I not have an undergraduate degree in psychology, but also my early college grades were horrid because I partied too much and had no direction whatsoever. I did find a school locally that offers a counseling degree and called to speak with them but I kept missing the director of the counseling program. I read in the catalog that one of the entry requirements was a 300 word letter of intent so I wrote one.

Letter of Intent

I would like the opportunity to earn my master's degree in counseling and fulfill my lifelong dream of being a therapist. My father was active in Alcoholics Anonymous when I was a child and began a support group for people with chemical dependencies. I was involved in his work at an early age and knew that one day I wanted to be a counselor too.

I have the ability to listen and communicate effectively and I possess strong people skills. I enjoy reading biographies and have always been interested in the behavior of people with extraordinary lives. I enjoy helping others. I have always been valued as a friend because of my confidentiality and ability to give "sound" advice. I am also capable of conducting small groups and classes and I am comfortable in a leadership role.

I value individuality, integrity, honesty, and love for my fellow man. I believe that we all are born with inherent gifts and abilities and we cannot be truly fulfilled until we are utilizing those natural talents. I believe that I have always been blessed with the personality traits of a good counselor but am now experiencing a life-altering illness that is pointing me in this direction professionally.

In June, I was diagnosed with cancer. I have been told since my diagnosis that I have a remarkable attitude and that others could benefit from talking with me about how I deal with having this disease. As I reflect on this I realize that it is an opportunity to redefine my professional future and utilize the experience of having cancer in a positive way. I believe that the time is right in my life now to return to school and work towards getting my license to practice therapy.

I would like to work primarily with people who, like myself, are facing a life-threatening illness and possibly establishing support groups to assist their families. As a supplement to this work I would also like to be available to work in conjunction with healthcare providers and/or public schools. I imagine this to be an "outreach" program whereby the counselor seeks the client, rather than the client seeking the counselor.

I believe the counseling profession would offer me a satisfactory income and enjoyable work environment, while allowing me to actively provide a valuable service to my community. In addition, I believe that counseling would allow me to best utilize my natural abilities, thus providing me with a personally rewarding career.

Betty J. Henson

Since my printer is not working, I went to Jim's office to print it. When I walked into his office, I noticed a picture of him and a woman on his desk. He tried to discreetly hide it but I saw him do it. He must be sleeping with someone. I was not surprised. On the way home, I had the urge to stop by the college. Although I didn't have an appointment, transcripts, or an application, I decided to stop in and just introduce myself.

When I got there, I was told that the Director of Counseling, Dr. Prescott was in and was available if I wanted to meet him. I was introduced to him and sat down in his office. He asked me questions about why I wanted to be accepted into the program. I told him that frankly, I wanted to become licensed and I needed my Master's to do it. He flipped through several pages of names and said; "All these people want to get into this program too, and I only have four seats left." We talked casually for a little while. He asked me what was in the folder I was holding. After he read my letter of intent, he told me that he was going to do something highly unusual.

He proceeded to tell me that he felt that going to graduate school would be very rewarding for me in light of my illness and that my experience would give me an edge over other therapists. He said that he had found out years ago that he had Parkinson's disease and so we were "kindred spirits". He told me a story about how he wanted to start a counseling degree program and the school was against it, but one man gave him a chance and now there are more students in the counseling program than in all the other programs combined!

He told me that he could not promise me full acceptance unless my undergraduate grades were sufficient, but barring that complication, he would give me a chance and take me as a student. I could have cried. He took me into the library and we were there for about two hours completing forms and questionnaires and before I left I had a complete schedule of my classes for the entire program. I feel I have encountered yet another "angel". There is something about this man that is very special.

If I am accepted and retain at least a B average, I will graduate in the spring of 2002 with my master's degree in counseling. As I got into my car to leave, I whispered a prayer of thanks to God for yet another blessing associated with cancer. When I got home I kissed my dad's picture and told him, "We're doing it daddy, we're doing it!"

September 5

I am sitting here in front of my computer with the most awesome sensation of "belonging" I have ever had. I feel like I have God's hand on my shoulder, guiding me. I do the same with the kids when we are in a crowded place. I don't push, don't hold tight, but just gently apply pressure to let them know that I am there and they are going in the right direction. Why do I do it? Because I love them and I don't want them to get lost or hurt. Because I want them to feel safe. Enough writing for now.

September 10

I had a follow-up appointment with Dr. Pollard last week. When he examined me, he was pleased. He said that under my arm previously was a "mangled mess" and that it had now become smoother with only a small palpable nodule. We talked about my upcoming surgery and he even cautiously hinted that I might not need more chemotherapy! I was so relieved to hear this, even though it may not be certain, it is some light at the end of the tunnel, a faint beam of hope that things may get better soon.

We talked a lot about the procedure of removing lymph nodes. I did not realize the extent or repercussions of this surgery until now. He said he would remove about 20 nodes from the first and second layers. This will remove the cancerous tissue there and also supply samples for pathology in determining further treatment.

The surgery will leave a scar curving around my ribs. I will experience pain and/or numbness and swelling in my arm and may not have full flexibility there. Some of this will be permanent to some degree. This is discouraging but it is a small price to pay if it means giving me a chance at a longer life.

My blood chemistry is a mess right now. My platelets, red, and white cells are all low. My white was the lowest it has been, at .2. Although I am getting my daily shots, I am not feeling the effects of them and I know they are not building my bone marrow back up as quickly as before. I have to be fully recovered from this before Dr. Pollard can operate on me.

I skipped writing about my last chemo session because it has been hard for me to even think about it. As I am typing this, I am getting nauseated, but I will proceed.
Jim wanted to go with me to chemo. He said that he felt it was his "right" since his insurance was paying for my treatment! Although I could really have a lot to say about that, I won't. The bottom line is that he wanted to go and so I decided to let him. I thought that if he saw what I had to go through maybe he would be more sympathetic. I also thought maybe it would somehow give him more of a feeling of involvement to help him feel like he was doing something for me. I really do want Jim to be okay. I don't want us to have a bad relationship.

When we got to the center, I went into the lab and was tested. This was the first time they had tested me prior to administration. My counts were too low and they would not let me have the chemo. Instead, I had to have shots. I was a little frightened by this, I must admit. Jim was chatty with the staff and witty with me and even though he said some things that unnerved me, it went okay. I was relieved. He even took me to lunch afterwards.

At lunch, I talked with him about wanting to go back to school. He told me he thought graduate school was a waste of money for me because of my uncertain future! All I could do was feel the sadness inside and not respond. I shouldn't have expected anything more from him. It was a typical response to something I really wanted to do.

He told me he would try to get me a portion of my settlement money as soon as possible because I need it very badly. All my bills are past due and I have no cash at all. Right now I owe Dr. Steinberg over 28 thousand dollars and still do not know if I will get Medicaid. I did hear from disability and I was denied.

Three days of shots followed with three days of pain, fevers, chills, and fatigue. My mood was low. I was depressed. On the last day, I was par for chemo and went in for my treatment alone for the first time since I started.

This day a new nurse administered my IV. She did not have a good bedside manner. She insisted on yapping about the drugs and how severe they were and how things could go wrong and of course they did. The IV did not drip. It was painful. The needle was against a valve in my vein and they were concerned that some of the Adriamycin leaked out into the surrounding tissue. I watched my hand get bright red. I was scared and I was retching inside.

Another nurse had to come and fix the insertion. I almost cried. The drip was slow and it was raining outside. I was cold and scared, sick and alone. I thought I would vomit before I made it to the car but I held out for several hours. Later that night I threw up for the first time.

The last time I had chemo I had done well to not depend on the steroids and instead was taking natural ginger tablets to cope with the nausea. This time I was violently ill. I got all my medications refilled and took them. For several days I was just plain sick.

Jim had told me he was going out of town Labor Day weekend and I assumed he meant he was taking the kids. I found out on Thursday before he was due to leave (the day after my chemo) that he was going alone (I later realized that he was actually taking his girlfriend that he had been seeing since March without my knowledge). I was shocked and panicked. I did not realize the kids would be with me and the fear of the upcoming weekend set in. He told me that his parents would be available to help but as it turned out, they were out of town too! I mustered all the strength I had and packed us all up to spend the weekend with my mother whom, by the way, had just been marked for her radiation and was in a weakened and ill state herself.

The day I was leaving to go to Mom's I heard kittens crying outside in the rain. I went to see about them and they appeared stranded. I brought them in. I found out who the owner was but he said he was looking for homes for them. I took them to my mother's and we gave them to the kids.

That weekend was really hard. The kittens kept the kids entertained but I was a mess. I was sick and weak. I went in and out of chills and fever and could not sleep at all. I was restless and could not get comfortable no matter what I did. Every time I thought about that IV I would get sick. I watched my hand turn blue and green. I heaved so much that I lost my voice for an entire day.

Finally through the weekend, I went back to the apartment with the kids. I felt some better and I decided to try and have at least one day with my children that I was not laying around sick. I should have used better judgment in retrospect, but I decided to take them on an inexpensive visit to the local zoo and a riverboat ride.

They had a really good time but the smells of the animals and the motion of the water kept me on edge and visibly stressed. I had to hold a paper towel over my nose the entire time to keep from vomiting. At one point I told them "Mommy is just too weak to keep walking and we have to go, I am sorry". They were wonderful and they understood.

The next day Jim came to pick them up and I was lying in the bed in a flannel nightgown because I was freezing (it was 90 degrees outside). I let him in and crawled back into bed. He talked to me later that day on the phone and said that he felt bad when he was here. I wasn't sure what he meant but he went on further to explain. He said that he wished I would make more of an effort to make myself presentable when I was around him! I was aghast. When he heard my reaction, he tried to say he thought my appearance scared the children. I lost control and totally cut loose on him. I cannot remember any of what I said except that I wish he had as much understanding and acceptance as they did.

Later that night I found myself despondent and lethargic. I wasn't aware of how I was sinking into despair. I picked up the phone to call my sister Bobbi. I wanted to cry and beg her to come and stay with me. I was afraid. I decided not to call her because it would only worry her. I got into my bed and didn't care if I ever got up. Nothing mattered to me at all. I knew that I could make the choice to get worse right then. I believe that if I had not been stronger I could have willed myself to die.

After lying in bed off and on for what seemed like days I picked up my dad's Bible and began reading. I don't know what I read or if the words even registered. I just knew I had to. I had tried to pretend to my online friends and people who called that I was fine but I knew I wasn't. I really felt like no one cared about me. Neither my family nor the man I had married and had children with. My heart was breaking that I had to go through this alone. During this time I asked God again to help me. I asked him to please take the burden of my sickness away and lead me back. I needed reassurance that God was with me if no one else was. I imagined Him to have big strong arms like my Daddy and that he would wrap me up in them and hold me. I held onto this image until I went to sleep.

I awoke the next morning to the brightest sunlight I have ever seen in my bedroom. It had been raining for so long I was used to the dullness in the morning. I got up and put on my clothes and just stood outside on the balcony. The air was cool and I decided to go for a walk. I couldn't go very far but it felt good. By that afternoon my spirits had changed. I had asked the Lord to lift me up and He did.

My next lab work showed my counts had dropped even lower. My body was not responding to the shots. I knew it because I had not felt the bone pains. But I was okay. I trusted God and I knew He would see me through. I did not let it get me down.

I have had shots now for the past five days. Five days ago I wrote the Sept. 5 entry in my diary. I could not write about all the horrors of the previous week at that time because it no longer mattered. The feeling I had of God being with me was so strong that it has been my only focus since then. Last night around 6 pm I experienced the most wonderful euphoric feelings I have ever felt. I cannot explain it at all. I just felt serene, peaceful, joyous, and happy. I felt like I was ALIVE.

Today I went to visit my mother. The kittens had scratched her hands and the scratches were getting infected so without hesitation I packed up the kittens and brought them back with me. I brought my mother with me and cooked dinner for her here. We talked a lot and she told me that she wanted to tell me something I would not believe.

She said that she knew some of the feelings I had felt the past week because she had felt them at the same time. I had not let her know all I was going through. She even called her sister on the phone to tell her that she was experiencing my pain. We talked a lot about the power of prayer. We had a very nice afternoon together and I felt good when I took her home. I believe this experience has not only brought my mother and me closer together, but it has brought us both closer to God at the same time.

September 11

I decided to write my half-sister another email. I had tried to let it go but I felt I was wrong in leaving it the way I did. I needed to tell her that the resulting loss of her relationship was not what I intended.

Just was sitting here thinking about you and wanted to write you. I am sorry about the way that I worded that last email to you, I truly am. I wish we could talk about this. I was on pain medication and feeling very much alone. I know, that's an excuse to you but it is the truth.

I know you feel that I was "ending" our relationship but that is honestly not what I was trying to do. (I was just fed up at the time and felt like you were just writing me out of obligation). I just wanted to be able to express some feelings that were bottled up...I meant that email for you and no one else...I blew out all those emotions at you but I didn't expect you to take it the way you did.

I sincerely had questions about all those issues I was telling you about, and still you haven't addressed any of them, so even though there is a rift now, I still don't know what to think about all that.

Whether you speak to me or not, whether we ever have any kind of relationship or not, it matters to me that things I have done in the past have caused you to be angry with me. I can't help it but I am just the type of person that if I cause those feelings, I want to know why so I can avoid them in the future.

You are my sister and whether we get along or not, it matters to me that somehow, in some way you can see some validity in my existence...that at some level I may have meant something to you or that you may have really cared. Nobody wants to feel like they are unwanted.

People can be very different but still make an effort at communicating if it is important.

Talking out of my head and of course I don't expect much of a reply (although one would be appreciated) but I just wanted to share this with you. And I would appreciate it if this would stay between us please? No sense in causing others to get upset over this when it doesn't involve them.

Thanks,
Betty

If nothing else is accomplished at all I hope for her to know that even though I was angry I do care about our relationship. I read over it now and it looks like I am begging her to show some compassion or love for me. This makes me so sad. What she chooses to feel about me is out of my control. Having sent this letter, I have decided to forgive the past. It is not important. I don't want to continue to rehash old feelings. I just want peace of mind. *(By the way, I never got a response)*

<u>September 12</u>

I have done well so far I think but I can feel this awful crying jag creeping up on me. I need a pity party to get it all out. I feel so terrible! I look like hell. My head is so pitiful. My scalp is flaking and peeling. My skin is very dry. Even on my nose and chin which has always had a tendency to be oily. The tears in my eyes are thick and they drain a lot. My legs and feet are swollen from the steroids. I feel bloated all the time. I have sores in my mouth and throat and a burning sensation all the way down my esophagus. The digestive problems have caused me to have painful bowel movements. The antibiotics give me yeast infections. I get dehydrated very easily. I have very little saliva and it is thick and mucous. Swallowing is difficult and I have to eat very slowly, taking small bites. I can only drink water because everything else either burns my throat, or is too sweet and makes me nauseated. I get winded easily and have very little energy. I have trouble walking across the parking lot to the grocery store. I have trouble carrying my groceries up the stairs. When I get inside, I have to sit down before I can get the keys out of the doorknob.

I wish people would visit me more. I wish instead of calling and asking what they could do that they would just think of something and do it. I wish my brother would call me and pray with me. He is a born again Christian and leads his church in worship but he won't call his little sister who has a life threatening illness. I just don't understand. I wish I could see Dill. I wish I were already through my divorce. I wish I had a better wig and felt like going to church. I wish I didn't have to worry about how I was going to pay my electric bill. I wish my children were a little more able to fend for themselves so I could spend more time with them. I miss them. I miss my dog. I miss my daddy. I miss having a house and a yard. I wish someone else would drive for a change.

I miss sleeping well. I miss waking up and feeling good. There is so much I want to do! I want to go camping. I want to go hiking. I want to see a waterfall. I want to see the mountains. I want to see snow. I want to run again. I want to sit in front of a fireplace and drink hot cocoa. I want to decorate a Christmas tree again. I miss my sister. I want my mother to be well. I don't want to go back to chemo. I don't want to have to go through radiation. I want to be healthy. I miss my hair. I just want to cry.

September 13

I feel like it is time to take a personal inventory of my journey since May. Where am I? Who am I? Have I accomplished anything? Have I learned anything? I have to look at my past first.

I had no direction in my life. I allowed my circumstances to determine my existence. I was either reactive or inactive and never proactive.

If things were not good for me, I felt sorry for myself or either I chose to blame something or someone for what I lacked.

I feel like I was a little shallow boat on some big body of water just drifting along with no destination, no maps, and no oars.

I would have glints of inspiration and spurts of motivation but nothing was ever substantial enough to move me to action or even belief.

Although I believe I have always been a loving person, I was selfish in my expectations. I always wanted love back and used it as a condition of giving it.

I didn't understand the concept of forgiveness. I allowed people to hurt me because I expected everyone to be sensitive to my needs. I did not allow people to be human.

I hid from myself because I didn't like who I was. I had no character. I had no backbone.

I had no identity. I always thought of myself as being open-minded and versatile, but I realize that I lacked commitment.

I have never summoned the courage to allow myself to believe in anything strongly enough that I would stand up and fight for it.

I have always been afraid of being wrong or being criticized. I have always been afraid of the shame and humiliation of failure.

How could I not see all this until now? What is it about seeing the end of your life so near that it allows such clarity about the past?

So what do I see in the present?

I am finding the inner strength I always felt I had but had never proven.

I am discovering the process of forgiveness and by doing so am freeing myself from past resentments to make room for more joy in the present.

I am learning that other people are human, that we all make mistakes, and that I am just as susceptible to failure as anyone else and therefore should not only be capable of accepting criticism, but of seeing it as a necessary part of my existence.

I am realizing that I cannot control other people and the way the feel about me or react towards me.

I understand how precious time is and how important it is to make the most of it. Making the most out of time does not mean doing more, but experiencing the fullness of each moment I am given.

I know that it is ok to have weak moments and to allow myself to release my anger and fear when I feel like I need to.

I am learning that I find most of my inspiration at 4 o'clock in the morning.

I know now that fear is more crippling than any disease.

I know that I am intelligent and capable and that my life is unique and valuable. I know that one person can make a difference.

I know that life is dynamic and it has natural periods of ups and downs. With those come success and failure, pleasure and pain, pride and humiliation, all worthwhile in the grander scheme of things.

I know that it is my sole responsibility what happens with this life I have been given. I do have choices that I can exercise.

I recognize the beauty and the power of love and I know therefore I am both beautiful and powerful because I have experienced it.

I am learning to be grateful for less and to show it more.

I am a unique and very special individual created by a wonderful loving God who wants me to be healthy and happy.

I know that feelings of happiness can be experienced in the midst of despair.

I understand that my battle is not simply against a physical death but also an emotional and spiritual one. Being alive is a gift! It has been given to me freely......but truly living? That is more difficult than dying.

I realize that I do not have all the answers and that is a good thing.

So what of the future?

I suppose the most awesome thing I am learning is that it is in the hands of God so I need not concern myself about it.

September 16

Last night I slept fairly well for the first time many days. My friend Toby flew in yesterday morning and I picked him up at the airport at 8:30 a.m. His hotel room wasn't ready until 3 p.m. so we came to the apartment to hang out while he was waiting to check in. It was the first day I had to spend all day without taking a nap or lying down and so I was exhausted.

I got invited to a baby shower, which is to be held tomorrow. I decided I didn't want to go wearing a baseball cap and so this morning the kids and I went to shop for a new wig. I found one that was very inexpensive that I liked. It is a shoulder length bob with bangs and is dark auburn like I used to wear my hair. I am wearing it now and it feels good.

September 21

This has been one of the longest days of my life it seems. I am scheduled for my node dissection surgery in the morning. I woke up early and got the kids off to school. I came home and lay down and ended up sleeping until almost 2 p.m. When I got up, I started cleaning since Bobbi will be here tomorrow for a couple of days. I guess I cleaned for an hour or so, got something to eat, and watched TV. I had a few phone calls and it was nice to hear from people who had remembered my surgery tomorrow.

It is 8:30 pm now and still dragging. I am anxious about tomorrow. I really don't want to have my underarm scarred like that but compared to a mastectomy it isn't that bad. I am tired of chemo and I don't want to have to do anymore of it! I am nervous about the pathology results. I want to be well. I want to get on with my life. I am tired of cancer interfering.

I am trying to prepare myself but I don't really know how. I think I will go take a bath.

September 25

Bobbi came over early Friday morning to take me to surgery. As we walked into the hospital, my name was called and I did not have to wait. I was taken immediately back into pre-op and prepped. There I met a male nurse named Duane who asked me if my chemo made me sick. I half-nodded and said "kinda." He said he understood because he had been there. I asked him what kind of cancer he had. He said he didn't have cancer but was exposed to Agent Orange in 1975. He didn't want to talk about it, I could tell. I just smiled at him.

I was taken into the operating room and my arms and legs were strapped down. I started to jokingly ask if I was going to be crucified and decided against it. Concerned, I told one of the staff that I wasn't groggy at all yet. He said, "I'm getting ready to change that." As he placed the mask over my nose he said, "Sweet dreams now."

I woke up in recovery with a huge bandage under my arm and a drain bag. Doctor Pollard came in and talked with Bobbi and I. He said he found some inflammation and scar tissue from the chemo. He told me to go see him Tuesday. Duane wheeled me out to the car and before I got out he squeezed and patted my shoulder. I understood what that meant. When you have battled cancer it enters you into an exclusive "society" of victims who all share the same fears, hopes, and emotions. You become brothers and sisters and there is a silent understanding. He was saying, "I fear for you, I hope for you, I understand."

On the way home I threw up in Bobbi's car three times, then again when I got inside. My mouth was dry from surgery and I had drunk a lot of water in the hospital in recovery so assumed that was the cause. Later in the day my nausea hadn't subsided and I also started itching all over and realized maybe I was having a reaction from the pain medication. I got out my pain pills Dr. Steinberg prescribed for my bone pain and started taking those instead. The nausea gradually got better. I had one of my "cold spells" where I started shaking uncontrollably, even though the apartment was about 80 degrees. I had told Bobbi about these before but this was the first one she had witnessed. She made an excuse to go to the store and when she came back, she had an electric blanket for me! She turned it on high and warmed up my bed before I got in it and I went to sleep pretty easily.

The next morning I was terribly sore. I rested a lot and took my pain medication as often as was prescribed. Bobbi helped me empty my drain and record the results. We watched several movies she had brought from home. That evening my mother-in-law called and we chatted for about an hour. She retired from the hospital after being a lab tech for 33 years. She asked me if they had decided to do a mastectomy and I said no. She expressed her disbelief about this and told me not to get my hopes up because she felt I would eventually have to have one. Talk about being negative! I hung up the phone and could feel the doubts and fears creeping up on me.

All night long I wrestled with feelings of depression and hopelessness. I kept telling myself that it was my previous telephone conversation that caused it and I needed to put those thoughts out of my mind. I read out of Daddy's bible and meditated before I went to sleep. I woke up Sunday and felt pretty good. I still had a lot of apprehension about getting my lab results and Bobbi and I spent a good deal of time Sunday talking about this. She had originally planned to leave Sunday morning but decided instead to stay until after I saw Dr. Pollard. I was glad because I really don't want to go alone.

Sunday night my bandage was itching and I was scratching my back with an unsharpened pencil. When I reached my left shoulder and upper arm it felt numb. Although I could feel the skin itching, I couldn't feel the pencil touching it. It was an eerie realization. I knew this was the loss of sensation Dr. Pollard warned me about. I tried not to panic, telling myself that the feeling would probably come back in time.

The bandage was crinkled up in the front and I pulled it off to try and flatten it out and when I did, I pulled off my skin in four places! It burned like crazy and I had to put ointment on it. I can't believe this happened.

I went to bed around 1 a.m. and slept through until about 11:00 a.m. I do not think I have been able to do this since I started chemo. I woke up a little hungry and feeling good. Jim came by the apartment to pick up a dress for our daughter's school pictures on Wednesday. While he was here he told me that his attorney had "put things on hold" until I progressed further with my treatment. I questioned this and he didn't have a reasonable answer for me. He left me confused and a little frustrated. I called my attorney and talked with her assistant. She made and appointment for me to talk to her tomorrow morning at 9:30 a.m.

I made myself get dressed and Bobbi drove me to run some errands. We went to the bank and I cashed a check. We then went to pay my electric and telephone bill. We got lunch at a drive-through and stopped by the post office and grocery store on the way back. By this time I was a little queasy. I came in and ate and then took a nap. When I woke up I started re-reading a book of my dad's on positive thinking.

I was impressed by the story of a young woman who had been diagnosed with terminal cancer. She had a strong will to fight and live and began using relaxation and imagery along with her chemo, imagining her white blood cells destroying the cancer in her liver. She also began focusing also on her life's goals and visualizing herself in the future, having overcome cancer and living the life she dreamed of. A subsequent test by her doctor showed that the cancer had indeed been eliminated. She attributes cancer to giving her a new direction in her life and helping her re-establish her priorities. These are the same feelings I have about my cancer experience and it helped me to be reminded of them.

I know for certain that my cancer diagnosis was the catalyst for positive changes in my life. I have reaped benefits of these changes already. I have experienced a much improved and enjoyable relationship with my mother, my sister, and my niece. I have been accepted into graduate school and am pursuing a career that excites me (for the first time in my life). I have begun to let go of the past, live in the present, and not worry about the future. I have put more trust in God. I believe that I will be victorious and this disease will be defeated.

"Who shall separate us from the love of Christ? Shall tribulation, or distress, or persecution, or famine, or nakedness, or peril, or sword? As it is written, for thy sake we are killed all the day long; we are accounted as sheep for the slaughter. Nay, in all these things we are more than conquerors through Him that loved us." –Romans 9:35-37

"God I know that you created me to be a healthy, happy individual. You have provided me with all that I need to have a long, fulfilling life. Although I am in desperate times now, I know that you are with me. I have faith that you will guide me through this darkness into the light of a new and better life. I believe that right now I am experiencing your divine healing and I thank you for it. Thank you also for allowing me to see the potential you gave me and for providing me the opportunity to achieve it."

September 27

Night before last I didn't sleep at all. I prayed and meditated when I lay down and lay in that meditative state for about two hours. At 7 a.m. I was still trying to drift off. Finally at about 9 a.m. I got out of bed to make coffee and woke Bobbi up.

I had a 9:30 telephone appointment with my attorney. I told her about Jim's nonsense comments. She explained it. He went to his attorney concerned that if he gave me money for school prior to the settlement being ordered that there was a possibility the judge would still deny the order because of my illness and he would be acting outside of a legal agreement, which could interfere with the repayment of that money. His attorney has had some conversation with her in which he expressed his personal feelings that I should be receiving alimony and because of my condition does not support Jim's actions.

I asked her if Jim's attorney would back down if we went to litigation and she said it appears he would. I asked her if that would free her to represent me and she said it would. I asked if she was willing and she said yes.

It seems that if Jim had any evidence whatsoever that he could use to pursue a lawsuit against me then his attorney would not be so willing to give up the case and be in support of me. I do not think he would be of the opinion that Jim should pay alimony if he had seen anything in Jim's files that would make me look bad. I have decided to get the money for school from Jim and then try to push this settlement through. One thing is certain: I am not afraid anymore of litigation. Bring it on.

I went to see Dr. Pollard at noon. The pathology report came back indicating that 13 out of 20 lymph nodes were positive for cancer. This is not the result I was hoping for of course but I was not shocked by it. I realize it is serious and that I will most likely have to do more chemo and perhaps maybe even more aggressive treatment than that. I am not upset or depressed by it. I am going to win this. I will do what the doctor tells me Thursday. I will give it all I have. I will get well. God is with me. I know it.

October 1

I am sitting here wearing my flannel nightshirt and a terrycloth turban. I look like a chemo patient. That's okay, because that is what I am right now. But I am a lot more than just a chemo patient. I am a 37 year old young woman with hopes and dreams and aspirations. I have just been accepted to graduate school. I have two beautiful children to take care of and people around me who love me. I look around me at the pictures on the walls and the "stuff" that surrounds me in the apartment. This is my home now. This place has been my shelter for the past nine months. I have laughed here, cried here, spent some of the loneliest nights of my life and yet some of the happiest.

The kids are playing their favorite game "kitty dragon" in the living room. They just got home from an evening out with Jim's parents. My mother-in-law called me earlier today and I told her that I was tired and still hurting from my surgery. She offered to take the kids out and I was happy. They had a good time. Tomorrow is an early morning for us so I am trying to let them wind down for a few minutes so they can go to sleep early.

They will watch cartoons until they get sleepy. Then I will go and tuck them in and kiss them and tell them how much I love them. I will take my pain pill and go to bed. I will meditate and sleep well. Tomorrow I will drive my children to school early and I will have a good day.

Saturday morning I was in a lot of pain and felt like I couldn't handle having the kids alone. I called Jim at 8 a.m. to see if he would make plans to pick them up that afternoon. He wasn't home. This was highly unusual because he has difficulty getting up early, even on weekdays. On weekends he sleeps very late. I continued to call, alternating calling his cell phone and home phone. Around 2 p.m. I realized that he simply wasn't home. At about 2:30 p.m. he called me. I could tell there was someone within earshot from his responses. I sensed he was with a woman. I asked him bluntly, "Where have you been?" He wouldn't answer me and changed the subject.

I told him that I didn't care what he did with his personal life but that I would appreciate it in the future if he would be more considerate. I told him that it hadn't been long since my surgery and he should have known I might need him and should have been more responsible about checking his messages because the children need to be a priority. He was apologetic. I cannot say I was very much surprised because deep down in my heart I knew he was sleeping with someone, but the thought of him having a relationship bothered me. It made me jealous. Not jealous of him, but jealous that he was able to be with someone else and I wasn't. In a way, I think Jim deserves to have someone else in his life. He has been through a lot, just like I have. But by the same token, I feel I deserve the same. I felt a surge of determination to beat this illness so I could get on with my life.

When Dill left to go back home the first week of July I assumed I would not see him for a while. I knew he had to go back to work and possibly go back to school in the fall. At first he expressed an interest in coming back down for the summer and finding an apartment and a job. He wanted to be close to me while I went through chemo. Although I wanted this very badly, I knew in my heart it was really not a good idea. Not only would there be possible complications because of my separation from Jim (I knew he would be furious and try to make trouble over it) but also I did not want my condition to keep Dill from doing what he felt like he needed to do in his own life.

I had hoped we could see each other again before he started school but it has just not been possible. I have not felt like I could drive that distance to see him and he could not afford a trip back down here. These past three months have been difficult without him. I miss him so badly. He is in school now and will not get a break until Thanksgiving. We have mentioned the possibility of seeing each other then but it will be difficult. It is too far for him to come down here during the time that he has off from school. The longest drive I have ever taken alone was 12 hours to go see my sister in Florida and at the time I was about 20 years old. If I drove 14 hours now I know it would be hard. Not only that, but I have a lot of feelings of self-consciousness about my appearance. I know it matters not to him, but I want to look better! I want to feel like doing things! I am going to have to make the decision to accept the way I am right now and make arrangements to go. I cannot stand the thought of waiting until Christmas vacation to see him.

Tonight I logged onto my computer and checked the date. I do this and have done this every single day since mid-January. I saw the word "October" and I thought, hey....I have been out on my own for 9 months. I have been through two surgeries and chemo for breast cancer…I am halfway through my treatment and damnit I can finish this. In twelve weeks it will be the end of the year. I can do this!

I went to see Dr. Steinberg Thursday. He told me that his hope is that the cancer was contained in the lymph nodes but even if it wasn't, I was getting the most aggressive treatment available and the chemo would destroy any microscopic cells in my body, aside from the breast tissue, which will be taken care of with the radiation. I am scheduled to start chemo again on Tuesday with Taxol. I will again go once every three weeks for four rounds. This will take me through December. Then in January I will do radiation therapy for six weeks. Following that I will go on Tamoxifen for five years.

October 6

Bobbi drove up Monday night and spent the night with Mama and then came over on Tuesday morning to take me to chemo. On Monday night I had to take 5 steroid tablets at 10 p.m. and then 5 more again at 4 a.m. I was afraid I would miss the 4 a.m. dose so I stayed up until after I took it.

When we got to the cancer center, it was busy. I had to go have lab work done. My blood counts were all good and so I went back into the treatment area. A new nurse started me and had a little difficulty with the IV but it wasn't bad. They gave me a whole bag of Benadryl. The Benadryl was to prevent a severe allergic reaction from the Taxol, like difficulty breathing. It made me weak and dizzy. The next drip was for nausea. The lab work and the first two drips took two hours. By the time the Taxol drip was started, I was already tired. I had a lot of trouble with my legs. I couldn't get them comfortable. I was ill and restless. The only thing I could do to tolerate sitting there for three more hours was to sort of wiggle my feet and keep shifting around. It was miserable.

Bobbi and I finally got interested in a couple of T.V. shows and it made the time pass by. I didn't feel any physical effects from the Taxol except a slight discomfort in my throat, like a tightening sensation. When we left, we went to eat lunch and then came back to the apartment. I was still woozy from the Benadryl but in pretty good shape. I could tell that the Taxol was not as hard on me as the Adriamycin had been. At least at that point.

The next morning we got up early and went out to eat breakfast. Then we went to visit my niece to see her new baby. As I cuddled and kissed her baby girl, I was saddened by the thought that I would never have another baby. We visited for about an hour, went shopping, and then came back home. She left to go back to Georgia and I lay down and took a nap.

Yesterday morning I felt stiff when I woke up. My joints felt swollen. I drank a glass of orange juice and noticed that my taste was gone again. As the day wore on, my back began to hurt and I ended up lying around most of the day. By nighttime, my body was aching terribly. I could not sleep all night. I kept getting sharp pains in my joints and in odd places, like my hands and my chest. The pains felt similar to the bone pains I get when my bone marrow is building up. I took a pain pill and lay back down.

I did not sleep much at all during the night. The pain in my legs, back, hips, and shoulders was severe. The sharp shooting pains were worse also and as soon as the cancer center opened I called and spoke to Lisa, the head nurse in the chemo department. She told me that I was feeling side effects from the Taxol. The sharp pains were associated with nerve endings and she advised me to take one of my Ativan nerve pills to help lessen that. The larger aches in my bones she explained usually appeared 48 hours after treatment and would be concentrated in my joints. She told me to take Norco for those. I took both medications.

I took a shower and got dressed but it was difficult. I had trouble getting in and out of the tub, drying off, getting dressed, etc. Several times it felt like my knees were going to give out on me. I was to pick up the kids today and needed groceries so I went to the store even though I did not feel like going. I was weak and stiff and had to move and walk slowly. I brought the groceries back home and put them away and then went to pick up the kids from school. The pain has been constant all day. Driving was stressful too because of the medication but I just took my time and used extra precautions.

I was so happy to see the children! I missed them. We went to the store to look for Halloween costumes and spent about an hour there. By the time we left I was exhausted but felt good that I had them and was able to get out. We came home and made tacos for dinner. After dinner I took more medication and just relaxed. I hope this will get better tomorrow. Getting up and down is hard and even just sitting or lying down is painful.

Today I called the Social Security office and asked how to go about appealing the decision to deny my disability. I also asked about the status of my Medicaid application. They are going to send me forms in the mail to complete and send back.

I also called Tina at the human resource office of the insurance headquarters. She remembered me. I asked her if I should just continue to wait to start working until I was completely through all treatment and she said yes. The position I was hired for was filled but she said at whatever point I am able to return to work they would see what positions are available at that time. The job hours are 9-6 and this would interfere with my Monday school schedule. Not only that, but the children's after school daycare closes at 6. If I do go to work there, I would have to work a different position where I could get off work by 5:30 at the latest. Although this may be a possibility, I am thinking I will be wise to look for something temporary with less stringent hours. I think I will call Sandy at the temp agency and talk to her. I had worked for them before. I would really like to start working in some capacity soon. I will wait first to see what the results of my appeal will be. If I am denied again, I think I will begin working right away, even if it is part time.

I have decided that instead of buying a mobile home I will try to find a house for lease. If I could find a house for sale with a lease purchase option, I could just make payments and not have to spend that money. If I could get one with three bedrooms and a yard for about the same I am paying here that would be nice. I do not want to spend my entire settlement on moving because I will need that money for school. Not only that, but I was told that my half-brother is having some problems with his landlord over his lease agreement on the land he and Mama live on. I do not think I want to place myself over there in the midst of a feud. If I have no choice left, I will consider it but only as a last resort.

Jim's niece Candy called me tonight. She is moving out of her mother's house and moving in with her boyfriend. I cannot believe this! Her husband is in agreement! That is outright adultery with cohabitation. I hope she realizes the danger she is putting herself in with custody of Tyler. She told me she has some furniture that she is going to give away and asked me if I wanted it. I am to go to the house on Sunday and look through everything. I think she has a table and chairs that I would like. I took the sofa and chair from the house and left Jim without living room furniture and Candy has a sofa and loveseat that she is giving away so I am thinking I will get that too for Jim. I want him to be able to fix the house up for Christmas for the kids. He told me tonight to come over one day and help him divide up the ornaments and such.

I talked to my attorney again this morning. Basically, I cannot afford to go to litigation and even if I did, because I was the one who left the marital home, there may not be much that I could gain above what is already in our separation agreement. I am going to ask Jim to continue to pay my car payments until I am able to pay them myself. I am also asking him to raise child support. I will not ask for alimony. I want my equity distribution to be available immediately. I am hoping that these changes will make the document more palatable for the judge. I believe I am ready to get some closure on this separation. I know I will not have enough money to pay my medical bills but they have told me I can pay as little as 10 dollars a month.

My biggest concern is being able to afford rent and utilities, and to pay all my tuition until I graduate. If I can get child support every month from Jim and have him keep up my car payments, then I can use a portion of the equity to cover the rest of my bills for the next year or so. During that time I can start working again. If I can find a house with a lease option to live in for the next year, then by the time the year is up I will have been working long enough to qualify for financing and should be able to purchase it. When I graduate I should be able to start working and making enough money I can begin to provide for us a lifestyle similar to what we had before. That is my goal, to move into a house, continue to go to school, start working after radiation, and try to buy the house at the end of the year.

<u>October 7</u>

Still fighting this nagging feeling of fear that keeps lingering just out of reach. I woke up this morning in tears. I was so scared. After Patrick was born I would get hip pains that the doctor told me were related to my pregnancy. After my daughter was born, I started getting back pains. I went to a chiropractor that told me my back was out of alignment from pregnancy and carrying my babies around. A couple of years ago I started getting uncomfortable stomach pains at night while I was lying in bed. It would start with my back and feel as if it were pushing through to my diaphragm. Now that I know I have had cancer in my body, I think about all those nights of aches and pains and I worry.

This morning I couldn't contain it anymore. My Uncle called. He is a pastor in a church in Florida. I was upset and I told him. He cried with me. He prayed for me on the phone. When I hung up, I lay there for a long time. I had a conversation with God. This is basically what I said.

"God, I have been trying to pray to you since all this started. I don't know if I am doing it right because I am now riddled with fear. I believe you are my creator and I believe you can help me. You have promised me that if I come to you with faith that you will provide for my needs. You have promised me that if I ask you for something in faith, you will give it to me. You have promised to help me defeat my enemies. You have promised me abundant life. Right now my biggest enemy is fear and I need you to help me defeat it. I am trusting you to pull me through this. I thank you for your love for me and your desire to bring me victoriously through this. I give this burden to you now."

Later in the day I began to feel better and have not felt like crying again.

<u>October 11</u>

This morning I compiled this letter to send to those on my email list:

Hello Everybody :)

Today I made the decision to participate in the [name] race on [date]. You may have seen the commercials on T.V. sponsored by the [name] showing women, some bald like me from the effects of chemotherapy.

This is only my second race. The first was the June, 2000 [name], also a 5K race. This is something I have always wanted to do and faced with the possibility I had cancer in May is what finally motivated me to enter for the first time. My niece completed the race with me, although we arrived late and missed "the pack" but ended up finishing anyway. Following that race, I realized that I could in fact make it to the finish line and wanted to try another one at some point in the future.

The reason I am writing all of you is because the race is more than just a fun day of walking/running. The [name] foundation is diligent in the search of a cure for Breast Cancer. If there was ever a need for this, it is now.

When I go to the center for my treatments, it amazes me how many people (young and old) are getting chemo. I have met many such wonderful people and had no idea just how many are affected by this horrible disease right here. It boggles my mind to consider how many there are in the Southeastern United States! Thousands of these people will be present in [city] to participate in this event.

This race is not just for victims of breast cancer but also for families and friends of victims. There are a lot of ways to participate besides actually entering the event. I would like to encourage all of you to check out the website for the foundation and consider whether you can contribute. If you are interested in walking with me, I would be deeply touched and honored to share this with you. The URL is [URL].

Please take a look at what the efforts of one woman with breast cancer can accomplish. Of all the lessons cancer has taught me, one of the most important is that each of us are valuable and one person CAN MAKE A DIFFERENCE. If any of you are interested in talking with me about this, please call me. The registration deadline for the race is October 13. If you choose not to participate then I would appreciate your prayers that I will be able to attend and better yet, MAKE IT TO THE FINISH LINE.

Wishing you health, love and peace!
Betty Henson

I had been nominated by members of the community to receive an award from a non-profit organization. They were having a fundraising meeting today and had invited me to sit in. Later in the morning I got dressed and went to meet the cancer fundraiser committee. The meeting was held at a fairly new restaurant that is owned by my cousin and her husband. I assumed she would be working but just in case she wasn't I sat down and wrote a note to leave for her.

When I got there I didn't see her. I found her husband and introduced myself. He said that she normally did work but today had a migraine and was home sick. I gave him the note and asked him to give it to her. A few people by this time were arriving for the meeting.

As it turned out, this was a planning meeting for the upcoming gala event they are holding as a finale to this year's work. The party will have a theme similar to the Academy Awards. Every table will have a top hat and gloves. Most people are dressing up like movie stars. There will be a formal dinner and dancing and they will hold a silent auction. The tickets cost 50.00 a piece and are tax deductible. The proceeds from the event will be given to the chosen local cancer victim(s). To my knowledge, there is only myself and one other woman.

I met her today. Her name is Destiny. When she walked in, my heart immediately went out to her. She was limping, in obvious pain. After the meeting we had a chance to talk. Her face and neck were covered with growths that resembled protruding marbles. She explained that her cancer started in the breast. She had a mastectomy and node dissection and later the cancer returned in the form of these tumors. She did not undergo chemotherapy or radiation! Since June, they have discovered 73 such tumors! I wanted to cry. She used to be a dancer. She has one son who is 17 years old and it is her hope to live long enough to see him graduate from High School.

Another woman I met named Linda was last year's award recipient. She was given ten thousand dollars by the committee to pay her medical expenses. She had undergone a mastectomy and chemo and at that time, her cancer was in remission. This April she began having back pains and went to the doctor. They did a bone scan and an MRI and found that the cancer had spread to her liver and spine. She has a metaport implanted in her chest and showed it to me. She has to go to chemo every week and will for the rest of her life, however long that is. Her treatments are over 5 thousand dollars a week. She was so negative. She insisted that when a biopsy is done, it "lets the cancer loose to run wild in the body". She complained about her doctors and her treatment. She had a sarcastic answer for everything that she was asked.

When I left there, I could tell that all those bad vibes were getting to me. I could feel the fear welling up and just keep thinking, my God, this is a horrible disease! I came home and checked my mail and had a bill for over a thousand dollars for my car insurance. I came into my bedroom, stripped out of my clothes, and went to bed.

As I was lying there I thought about how often in the beginning I retreated to my bed as an escape. I have done this less and less as time goes on. Early on I would just go to bed and sleep for long periods of time to pass the time away, waiting for things to get better. I realize now that things don't get better with inaction. I eventually got up and started cleaning house.

Soon my life is going to be full of accomplishments. Next week I will start back to school. In two weeks I will be walking in the Charleston Race. Soon after will be Patrick's birthday party, then Thanksgiving. Before I know it, it will be Christmas and then New Year's, then time to move, finalize the divorce, and start working again.

October 12

This morning I had nothing to do and was wondering how I was going to spend the day. The phone rang and it was my mother, wanting me to take her shopping for a pair of shoes. I got dressed and went over there. She was supposed to meet me at 1 pm following her radiation treatment but she wasn't there. While I waited, I began walking. I think I walked about two miles.

When she got home we went out for lunch and then to the shopping center. She bought a pair of shoes and I bought a winter jacket and bathrobe. When we left we went by a consignment shop to look for a formal dress for me to wear to the banquet. A woman was there, nicely dressed and made up and chatting about all the clothes she has that she doesn't wear. She made the comment to the clerk that "we women always have too many clothes, but can we really resist?" I thought to myself how shallow this sounded and yet how wonderful it would be to have my biggest worry to be what I was going to wear.

Cancer invades your rational thinking. It saddens you. It makes you wish you had done more in the past. It makes you consider your mortality in every thing you do. It makes the future seem so uncertain. It is a disease of the mind as much as it is a disease of the body.

I have been asked to address the audience at the fundraiser banquet. I have no idea what to say except I know that I don't want it to be dreary. I want to say something that shows my attitude of hope and determination. I think I will pull excerpts out of my diary and maybe add a poem.

October 15

Had a full weekend. On Friday I went to physical therapy. I was so impressed. My arm was so stiff I couldn't straighten it but by the time the therapist was finished I was relaxed and had full extension in my arm. I went shopping afterwards before picking up the kids from school and tried on winter clothes. Then the kids and I went to the bookstore and stopped by a pizza place on our way home.

On Saturday I took them to play miniature golf and then we went out to eat and they played on the indoor slide. Saturday afternoon they met some kids outside the condos here and played with them, and then today we went walking first thing. We checked out the hotel lobbies in the area for about a mile and picked persimmons off a tree in the neighborhood. Later we went shopping for pajamas, went to eat lunch, stopped by the grocery store, and then came home. We just finished eating soup I made and they are about ready for bed. I am tired but happy that I was able to keep them busy all weekend and keep up with them!

I have noticed that my mood seems to be much better now. I am getting back to the point I was at before when I wasn't thinking about cancer as much as I was just trying to enjoy my life. I have a busy week ahead (therapy three days and start school tomorrow!) so I am hoping this will keep my focus elsewhere.

I talked with Dill about Thanksgiving week and his mom said that I would be welcome to stay there if I wanted to visit. He was teasing me about having to bundle me up like an Eskimo while I was there. He can't believe that I am in South Carolina and am using an electric blanket! I probably will freeze but I don't care! I am really excited and looking forward to going up. I can't wait to talk to Dr. Steinberg and find out if it will be possible. The time I am planning to go falls right on Day 8-14 following my chemo, which is normally the time I am in the office getting daily shots. I hope this will not be the case but I will just have to wait and see.

<u>October 16</u>

Revelation: been depending on treatment to cure me and not totally convinced it would...just realized that I have an immune system given me by God to get rid of this cancer and if I put faith in my immune system and Him I will get well...chemo is just to help kill the cancer faster so my immune system can handle it and I have to believe it will.

<u>October 22</u>

Today is a beautiful day; warm and sunny, not a cloud in the sky. I woke up this morning and went for a long walk in the neighborhood. As I walked past houses and apartment buildings, I saw people going about their lives...one woman piling up leaf clippings by the roadside, a couple in a new house arranging new shrubbery in the yard, a young man sitting on his porch listening to music, an older gentleman walking his dog, two children playing in their courtyard, and an older couple arriving at a house to visit someone.

I look at them with different eyes than I used to. I don't see perfect families living perfect lives anymore. I see individuals coping with life and trying to enjoy themselves in the process. I realize that I have no idea the struggles others are going through but that they do exist. In the past I wanted to trade lives with these strangers. I could wish for that now to escape my illness, my economic hardship, my pain. But I don't. I know that my life is unique and I am going through rough times that are a result of choices I made in the past.

I really believe that cancer invaded my body because it was so weakened by stress. The stress of my childhood memories, the family unhappiness, the powerlessness I felt in my own life, my insecurities, the marital difficulties I experienced, and the lack of taking good care of myself. By the same token, I believe that I can overcome cancer by eliminating all of that stress. I have accepted that my past wasn't great but it is over and done with and doesn't matter anymore. My financial problems will get better in time, when I am able to go back to work and have a more stable income. The divorce is only three and a half short months away. I am trying every day to take better care of my body. I am giving it vitamins and minerals, more water, more fresh air, better food, and exercise. I am getting the best medical care available and I am incorporating mental techniques to help me achieve a higher level of spiritual wellness. I believe I am taking an active role in fighting cancer.

I am trying to enjoy the present more. Every morning I wake up and fight the urge to lie around and contemplate my circumstances. All that does is create worry and negative feelings of helplessness. And in the meantime, life goes on around me, without me. I have made the choice to not let this happen. The world exists for my pleasure as much as the next person's and it is up to me to indulge in it. Yes, there is a lot I wish I could change. I'd like to hurry things along, hasten my divorce, end these treatments so I can work again, move right now into a better house, but the time is not ripe yet for those things. Those are things I cannot change and I have to accept that for now and try to make better the things I can change.

I have started graduate school and am enjoying my classes. I have met some interesting people and have gained an amazing amount of insight into my own personality already as a result of the information I am learning. The academic challenge is exciting. I am not approaching it with the sense of dread and fear that I once did when I was in college. I see it as an opportunity to stretch myself, to grow and become more knowledgeable, more capable, more developed intellectually. I embrace it.

Last night I attended the fundraising banquet. The girls had put together a wonderfully elegant affair. I sat and watched the guests arrive. The men were donned in tuxedoes and black ties and the women in gorgeous sequined gowns. I admired the hair mostly (not surprising). I sat with Destiny and her roommate Carol and we mused about the irony of the situation. People came over and hugged us and spoke encouragement and support and we smiled and pretended to have a marvelous time but the truth was that we would rather have been anywhere but at a charity ball to honor us as breast cancer victims.

I talked with her more intimately on a trip to the ladies room about her condition. She was hospitalized for two weeks recently because of a bowel obstruction. During her tests it was discovered that the cancer had also invaded her liver and her doctor gave her a 6-months-to-live scenario. This infuriated me. How does he know? No human being has the ability to determine when any of us are going to die. Why take away her hope? What is the point in trying to be realistic when you are only considering past case histories and statistics? I refuse to let numbers in black and white predict the outcome of my life! I am not a statistic and I don't ever want to be treated as one. I'll be damned if anyone will tell me when I am going to die and if for some reason they try, I'll be sure to prove them wrong because it is so absurd!

Last night I woke up with the urge to read out of Daddy's bible. I picked it up and turned to a page randomly and found some passages he had highlighted. They referred to the conflicts between the flesh and the spirit and how we have a choice to allow ourselves to either be ruled by our bodies or by our creator. My body is under the power and authority of my spirit that is led by God and therefore it must obey. No matter how bleak my prognosis may appear it is an opportunity for the spirit to triumph when my complete healing is confirmed.

My thoughts are constantly tugging at me. There is this underlying power struggle between feelings of being helpless and victimized by a disease that could end my life and feelings of being on a divine journey that could have a joyful outcome. I don't want to be restricted by the "realness" and danger of cancer yet I don't want to be in denial about it either. I have tried to find a median place where I can accept the fact that I am fighting a life threatening disease while holding on to the hope that I will be able to defeat it. It is maddening at times. One thing I am clear about though is that no matter what, I have to remain determined to fight. The weaker I get and the more helpless I feel, the harder I have to work to summon that fighting spirit but I believe it is the most important thing I can do above all else.

October 23

I sent the following to the people who are closest to me, the ones I can trust with my deepest feelings, and others that I believe could be touched by knowing what I am dealing with. Perhaps I did it to explain my irrational behavior at times, or maybe even as a way of crying out to them. I recognize the importance of allowing my feelings to surface. When I hold it in it seems to eat away at my spirit, so I am letting it go. Although I have expressed these feelings similarly in previous journal entries, this time it was meant to be shared.

What it's like to have cancer...

You hear the ugliest three words of your life. They can vary from "It was positive," or "I was right" or "It was cancer," or "I am sorry," but they all have the same meaning- your descent into hell itself. The times ahead will seem like an endless roller coaster ride with hills and valleys, each successive high a little lower than the one before.

In the beginning, you feel fine. You look "normal". You tell yourself, they can cure me, I am strong. But as the days turn into weeks and the weeks turn into months, the reality sets in. The professionals are kind and caring and they tell you that you are doing great, but you think "compared to what?" You read the statistics on cancer and you begin to realize that the figures are not on your side but you tell yourself you are more than just a number on a page.

You search for small glimmers of hope in places you never looked before. You read lots of books written by survivors that tell you what to eat, how to pray, where to go for help. You try music therapy and vitamins and herbs and yoga. You listen with solemn gratitude to every person who offers you encouragement but words cannot cure you.

Nothing about your life remains normal. You shop for clothes and you wonder why new clothes are necessary when you have no hair. You buy groceries and you wonder, should I continue to eat preservatives and additives with carcinogens. Every smiling person you meet seems to mock you. You long for the days when your smile was a genuine one that wasn't a screen for the desperation you feel inside.

You think about the past and how you wasted so much time. You think about the future and wonder if you will be part of it. You worry about things you haven't done or things you did do that you shouldn't have. Then the fear creeps in. You lie in bed at night and feel discomfort in odd places and suddenly you realize that you have felt this discomfort for years. Then your body gets flushed and you get scared. What if the cancer is there too? And you cry in mourning for the person you once were.

All the while you try and devise ways to keep from being depressed, to keep the wolves at bay. You crumple bad thoughts up like paper and throw them out. You stuff them in black balloons and you send them floating away. Trying to stay positive takes all your energy, especially when you encounter cynical or thoughtless people. They are the ones, for example, that tell you a story about someone they knew who had cancer and even though they died, they lived a good life, like it should make you feel better.

And you get angry. People who love you try to comfort you and you hurl insults at them. You are denied coverage by the insurance company and you call them and raise hell. Your VCR decides to eat a tape and you beat it to death. You read books by the so-called experts that say anger is good, get it out, but in the process you risk burning bridges that you don't know if you have time left to re-build.

The nights are incredibly lonely. You wake up in pain and there is no one there to comfort you. You yearn for someone to hold you and the space where their arms should be is empty. You want to be a baby again, to be innocent and ignorant of the danger that lurks around you. You know that the path you are walking is a dark one and you don't know where it will take you but you keep moving forward because you have no choice.

At times, you feel alive and you want to be part of the world around you. Though it's hard to mingle with the "living" crowd, you do it anyway and for awhile it makes you feel good until the party is over and you take off your wig and see the bald head of chemo staring at you in the mirror. You've been initiated into a society of victims that you never applied for membership to. You want to escape but there is none.

And every once in a while, you experience joy and it takes the disease away momentarily. The kiss of a child, the beauty of a sunrise, or just a funny movie that makes you laugh until your sides ache. But then you get sad because you know that it is only temporary and that the fears will return. So you brace yourself, armed with only your mind.

Through it all, you are determined to remain steadfast, to fight it, to beat it, against the odds. You know that your best ally is your attitude but it doesn't seem to want to cooperate. The medication makes you tired and if you can sleep, you dream about invisible attackers out to get you. The chemo makes you sick and you don't like throwing up but you have to go back, day after day and willingly allow another poison injection. You try to envision your body getting well but it has been so long since you felt good you don't really know how.

And people say, "one day it will be over and you will be fine," and oh, how you want to believe this. You repeat over and over like a mantra, "I will get well, I will get well," hoping something in your subconscious will pick it up and act on it. And you talk to God a lot. You bargain with him at first and then realize how infantile it is to bargain with God. You pray and you summon all the faith you can muster and for a while it gives you peace.

Crazy thoughts enter your mind even though you don't invite them. You find yourself thinking, "if things get bad enough, I have that bottle of valiums in the medicine chest", but then you snap out of it because you realize that you have responsibilities and commitments to the people who love you and depend on you to be okay. You have to keep going because you don't want to hurt them but every time you look at them you want to cry. You want to be there for them, more than anything in the world but you don't know what to do to make that happen. You are powerless.

There is really no one you can be totally honest with. People want to listen but they don't really understand because they haven't faced it. The ones that try the hardest are the ones that truly care but they are the very ones that you don't want to be negative around. And then there are those that cannot rise above their own dysfunction to even pretend they care because they don't know what to say or worse yet, something they say may embarrass them, God forbid, so they don't contact you.

You try to find some deeper meaning in the experience. You hold on to the belief that something inherently good will surface out of the tragedy of it all. You envision all the dreams you've ever had coming true and how the course of this horrid disease could lead to victory. While you hope you wait, battling the demons along the way. In the process, you learn to live in the present. You let time creep along as you struggle to keep your head above water so you don't drown in your self-imposed misery. You squeeze the most out of every day even though it leaves you exhausted in the end but the fatigue helps you collapse into that glorious unconscious state where thoughts can't steal your sanity.

And every once in a while, you wake up to a bright sunny morning and you feel good. Your expression is one of a person who has wisdom brought about by heartache. You reach out to others because you feel like you have something to offer. You want to make your mark on the world and you feel like you can. You hold the bittersweet knowledge that the only day any of us has is today and so you forge ahead in hopes that you will be granted another day like the present one.

You experience compassion you didn't know you had. You find yourself acting as a messenger of hope. You want to give to others what you need yourself. You break through barriers of incompetence and weakness that used to stifle you. You feel the seeds of greatness sprouting from within and you know that your journey will forever change your outlook on the world. For the moment you are important, powerful beyond measure because by staring death in the face you are learning to live. You know you will never be the same, regardless of the outcome, and so you watch it slowly unfold, with all its pain and glory, your life with cancer.

October 25 (Daddy's birthday)

I went to the cancer center yesterday for my treatment. After he examined me, I talked with Dr. Steinberg about the problems I am having that I have only recently begun to pay attention to. I told him about the soreness in my right rib, the burning in my stomach, and the throbbing pains in my knees and shins, and my backaches. I explained to him that most of these symptoms started over 4 years ago after my daughter was born and that I had felt some fear now that it could be related to the cancer. He said if it would ease my mind he would order a bone scan and Aubrey got me an appointment for November 6. Although this is what I thought I wanted at that moment, I decided that I am not going to go through with it.

I have to believe that my body is now cancer-free. I have three more months of treatment to go through, while tackling my classes and taking good care of my children. I have to find a house to live in and move at the end of the year and then get moving on the divorce in January and possibly buy a more economical car. I just have too much to be concerned about already. I have been holding onto the vision that by February I will be cured and can move forward with my new life. This has given me the motivation to endure these treatments, the pain, the loneliness, and the poverty. If I were to find out that my illness was more extensive, I don't think I would have the will to get me through all I have to do at the beginning of next year. When things calm down and I have my life in order then I will consider the test. All this was on my mind as I waited to start my chemo.

Bobbi was running late and while I waited for her I chatted with a lady named Margie. She was an attractive older woman with a sweet smile and she appeared nervous and apprehensive. I found out it was her first treatment and she didn't know what to expect. She had breast cancer several years ago but has been in remission. The doctor recently found a spot on her lung but said it was unrelated to her breast cancer. She was getting Taxol also so I tried to prepare her for what it would be like.

We chatted a bit and then Bobbi showed up and we were both started on our IVs. Bobbi had accidentally left her wallet on top of her car and drove 10 miles before she noticed credit cards flying behind her in the rear-view mirror! She spent 45 minutes walking along the highway retrieving the contents of her wallet but miraculously found everything except her Cross pen!

I had another new nurse and, as is becoming the norm, she had trouble with my IV. She stuck the needle in wrong and couldn't get a good blood return. I was wincing, in pain. I thought she was going to cry but I tried to calm her down and convince her that I was okay. Peg (I affectionately call her "Tiger Lady") took over and got the line in properly. I had forgotten to take my Decadron the night before so they gave me a drip.

Then came the Benadryl, 50 mg. I told Jennifer that it typically made me woozy and she suggested that if it did, next time I should try 25 mg. I got so dizzy I thought I was going to pass out. I couldn't look out the window because the trees were fuzzy and moving in squiggly patterns. I had to hang my head and cover my eyes to get through it, but after about 15 minutes it began subsiding.

The Zofran caused me to have "fanny burn" for the first time. This is a reaction that hits suddenly in the lower torso and feels like burning, stinging insect bites in the buttocks and genitals! It was highly uncomfortable (I hesitate to call it pain but I suppose it was) but it didn't last very long, maybe 2 or 3 minutes.

The Taxol went smoothly and I didn't feel any discomfort except that my hand got so cold I had to bundle it under two blankets.

Bobbi and I talked and had a lot of catching up to do so the time passed very quickly. Dr. Steinberg came in to get a drink of water and stopped and chatted with us. I asked him about leaving town the week of Thanksgiving and he said it was a good possibility. This made my day! I am really looking forward to going to New York and visiting Dill and meeting his family. I think the change of scenery will be beneficial to me and I know spending time with him will lift my spirits tremendously. I am excited about going!

With so much to talk about, the five hours of chemo passed quickly, unlike the last time. We left and went to eat lunch and then came back to the apartment. I was tired and still groggy from the Benadryl so Bobbi went to the grocery store for me while I rested. She spent the night again and we stayed up until about 2 a.m. I went to sleep around 3 and didn't wake up at all until this morning around 10:30!

I got up and drank a cup of coffee and then got dressed and we went to eat lunch. We had a nice time. The only problems I had from the chemo were a burning sensation in my face (it even looked bright red like sunburn) and loss of taste, which I guess will be the rule now until the end of my treatments. After lunch, Bobbi had to get on the road to beat the rush hour traffic in Columbia so she left right away.

Although I was tired by then, I knew that I had to go follow up on my Medicaid application and my Disability Claim Appeal. I went to the Department of Social Services and was promised that my Medicaid would start this week and be retroactive for 90 days. I am so thankful for this! My medical bills are now up around 38 thousand dollars and this would cover all but about 2 thousand!

I didn't have the same luck at the Social Security office, however. If my appeal is successful and I am granted disability, it will begin paying 6 months from my date of disablement, which was around the end of June. That would put my benefits starting December. I will not even get a response for about 90 days so even if I can get it, it would only help me for two months. If I get it I will be grateful but I am not counting on it.

When I got home this afternoon, I had a message on my answering machine from someone I hadn't had contact with in years. It was a girl I was friends with in High School. Her mother goes to church with my sister-in-law and heard her ask for prayer for me, found out what I was going through, and told her daughter. I called her back and talked with her for over an hour.

As I hung up the phone, I could tell my pelvic bones were starting to ache and I knew to get prepared for the side effects from the Taxol. I took a pain pill and sat down in front of the computer. I chatted with Dill for about an hour and then he called me and we talked for another hour. By this time it was midnight but I wasn't sleepy so I started this journal entry. Now I am having pain in my hips, legs, back, and breastbone. I am going to take another pain pill and try to go to sleep.

October 29

The past several days have been rough. I have been in awful pain, taking pain medicine and nerve pills, overlapping them at times. I had one day that was particularly bad and had to go to the store and almost couldn't make it back up the stairs. Most of the time I just lay around watching TV. I did a lot of homework and reading. Even though I was in pain and felt really bad, I didn't cry about it. I have only had a few phone calls. Jim, Dill and my mother have called to check on me.

Friday night I knew that I couldn't walk in the Charleston Race. I was hurting too badly and could hardly walk to the car. I was bummed about missing it but I knew I had to. I needed to rest. The kids are with me and we have been taking it easy. I cooked dinner for them tonight (beef stew and noodles) and they loved it. I am always pleased when they eat well after I have cooked for them. It gives me a lot of satisfaction.

Last night I chatted with Jim. I opened up to him and for the first time in a long time, he took the time to listen to me. I told him that I was sorry for hurting him. I told him that I no longer blamed him for the things that went wrong in our marriage. I told him that he was a wonderful father and that I loved him for that. I told him I wanted us to always be close and that I wanted him to be happy.

Tonight I have been sitting here listening to one of my favorite CDs and have felt pretty good. I am still hurting but it's not so bad now. I have done a lot of thinking about my life over the past year. So much has changed! I am not the person I was a year ago.

I have learned a great deal about myself and I am pleased at what I see. I have accepted that I have a terrible illness but I am hopeful I will overcome it. At times I have found myself in a position of waiting until it's all over but I realize that I cannot do that. My life is important right now and I don't have to wait to enjoy it. Every night that I lie down to go to sleep after having a productive day I feel good. I don't have to live according to any one else's standards anymore. I don't have to please anyone. I only have to feel like I am doing my best. And I am.

I am proud of myself. I have become a strong, courageous woman. I am facing the difficulties in my life with the belief that I have what it takes to overcome adversity. I have become more confident in my abilities. I am no longer as self-conscious about the way I look. There is a much more beautiful self inside that is becoming more apparent as days go by. I have a huge capacity for love. I know that when I love, I love deeply and spiritually.

I have this inner knowing now. I feel more connected to the universe and to life itself. I am feeling at peace. I am not worried about the future. I know that my needs will bc met. I have more faith in God than ever before. I know that he will see me through. I want to live. I want to watch my children grow up. I want to be available for them. They are so precious to me. I am depending on God's grace and mercy to sustain me. He loves me. He is good. He will provide.

<u>October 31</u>

Have run myself ragged the past two days. Started both days at 6 am getting the kids ready for school. Yesterday took breakfast and coffee to my mom's and starting reading the classifieds, looking for a house. Ran a bunch of errands paying bills, etc., took my mom shopping and to the pharmacy, bought groceries and cooked dinner at her house, ate with her and the kids, visited with my brother and his granddaughter and got home about 9 pm. I was beat.

Then today came home and napped after taking the kids to school. Got up and went to Dr. office and got my CBC. Much to my surprise (and delight!) my counts were all above normal! I was sooo happy! I told them I wanted to go out of town over Thanksgiving and was hoping to avoid shots that week so I could go and they teased me, wanting to know where I was going, who I was going to see, etc. They were all dressed up for Halloween and it was a fun visit. I have gotten to know the staff pretty well and I always enjoy talking to them.

I went to a real estate office afterwards and talked to the broker my sister used to work for about my situation and wanting a house. Even though it is a long shot that I will be able to buy one, she told me they had done it before and not to worry about it. She gave me a list of houses in my price range and one of them was a house I have driven by several times and thought would be perfect! It has 3 bedrooms, 2 baths and a fenced-in yard in a decent neighborhood near my mother and close to the kids' school and the job I was hired for. Again, I felt like God was there. I believe he has a plan for me, much greater than I could have imagined for myself. There is a house out there somewhere that he wants me to have and I just have to keep looking until I find it!

Later, I dressed the kids up in their costumes and we went trick-or-treating. They had a really good time. It was fun and sweet and I enjoyed being out but of course walked a lot and got really tired. I drove them over to Jim's parents' house for a brief visit and then picked up dinner at a drive-through and came home. Again, another night of getting home after 9 pm….exhausting but exhilarating.

I have a big school project I have to be ready for next Monday and I need to get my butt in gear and get ready for it. I will take tomorrow to study and may make an appointment to look at that house but otherwise I am going to take it easy. The kids will be with me until Thursday morning and then Jim is going to pick them up. I will have lots of time through the weekend to rest and do my research.

I stopped in at my landlord's today to pay my rent and talked to him about the kittens. The owner of my unit is adamant about not having pets and so I was advised to do something about them. I have no idea what I will do. Maybe I can move soon. Maybe Mama can keep them again. Maybe they can stay with Jim for a couple of months. I don't know what to do. I can't get rid of them. The kids love them to death and I won't take them away. Another thing for me to worry about! But I believe something will work out.

In one hour it will be November. November! It has been one year since I started thinking about leaving my marriage. This time last year I was oblivious to the cancer that was growing inside my body. I never considered my mortality. I took so much for granted! What a pitiful state I was in! If I had been diagnosed with cancer then my outlook would be so darkened and desperate! I can at times imagine what my life would be like now. I would still be in that house, living constantly with a man that didn't show his appreciation for me. I would feel so helpless and despondent. I know I would be terribly depressed. I know I would not have as strong a will to live as I do now. Thank God for his impeccable timing!

I believe I had to have those months of being on my own to regain my confidence and to get excited about my future in order to prepare me for the task ahead and give me the strength to endure it alone. I learned in that short period of time that I could take care of myself financially. I learned to pay my bills on time and balance my checkbook I learned how to pass the time without constant companionship and depending on another for security.

It could be that if I had detected the cancer earlier, my "statistical" chances for recovery would be much greater but I don't think my desire for recovery would be as strong. I think about how that time may have made a difference in the severity of my illness but I still believe that it has happened the way it was supposed to. God's will again. He has lifted me out of my despair and set me on a path that will lead me to true happiness. I thank him for it!

I have been stripped to my core. All that was my old life is gone. I lost my job (which I disliked), my financial security (which was based on my husband's accomplishments), my "mate" (whom I never felt really loved or understood me), my home (that I despised), my daily routine (which I always considered to be unfulfilling). Thank God for exposing in his mysterious ways what is truly important- ME!

Daddy used to tell me that sometimes we have to be lying in a ditch, flat on our backs in order to see the stars above us because when we are upright we don't look in that direction. He was so right. All I could see then was the periphery…those around me, living lives I wished I had, basing my wants and desires on earthly possessions and I saw only what I lacked. Lying on my back now I see so much more! I see the beauty of life and the potential happiness that I know exists within me. I am more detached from worldly things and more attached to my creator. I am more dependent on Him and more trusting.

Now that I am down to the point where all I have is me, I have the chance to start over, rebuilding myself from a stronger foundation. As daddy used to say in his speeches with Alcoholic's Anonymous, "you have to sometimes hit rock bottom before you can begin the climb to success". He was a brilliant man with such insight into life. I am thankful I had so much time with him to learn from him.

I talked with Dill tonight and he gave me some sound advice (as he always does). He said that we all have fears related to our circumstances and regardless of what they are, we can choose to give them power over us so that they manifest in our lives, or we can refuse them. I do not want fear to control me!

November 3

I just got back from Dr. Steinberg's office. I called to cancel my bone scan yesterday and as soon as I hung up the phone, Audrey called me back to find out what was going on. I talked to her about it. She is going through a similar situation as me; marital separation with two young children, struggling to pay her bills, etc. I told her that I was alone and if the diagnosis wasn't good, I didn't know if I could deal with it. She encouraged me to talk to Dr. S about it. We made an appointment for this morning.

I have a big project for school due tomorrow morning. I haven't been able to concentrate on my work. All I could do since yesterday was cry. I ended up totally stressed out by night and had a splitting headache.

I turned off all the lights in the apartment and lit my candle on the dining table and sat down with my rosary. After praying my rosary, I was sitting there with my eyes closed and I clearly heard a woman's voice call my name. I turned to look towards the kitchen, where the voice seemed to come from and there was nothing there. Then I noticed out of the corner of my eye a shadow, like the outline of a woman's head against the wall. I looked there but it was gone. I said, "I heard you but I don't see you"

Then I saw a bright red flash of light coming from the corner of the room. I looked directly at it and watched it, hovering in the air, flickering, then fading. I felt like I was seeing an angel, or a spirit of some sort. While it was there I had the most peaceful feeling! Even after it disappeared I knew the presence was still there. I did not feel alone. I said to God, "please make it come back", and I heard a silent response in my head saying, "Be still and know that I am God," (when I was building my website, I found a graphic that looked very much like the light I saw and behaved in the same manner. I put a cluster of them in and they are programmed to follow the cursor. If you are interested in seeing the image, it is at www.onlinecounselor.info).

I had felt alone and God had sent me company. I felt that he was telling me that he would provide for my needs and that I only needed to concern myself with the present moment and he would give me what I needed at that moment. I immediately thought to call Bobbi and tell her but I wasn't sure if I should. I asked God, "do you want me to tell others about this, or should I keep it to myself?" and I got the feeling that he wanted me to share it.

As crazy as this all sounds, it was a real experience. I called Bobbi and told her and she said that when the phone rang, she was praying for me. We talked for a few minutes and then I went to bed. My headache was gone and I did not feel any pain anywhere in my body. I went to sleep easily and soundly.

I broke down into uncontrollable tears again this morning while I was getting dressed. I tried to calm myself down before I got to the cancer center. I am usually upbeat and talkative and I didn't want to go there with my eyes swollen and face red from crying.

In the waiting room I ran into Margie, the lady I met at my last chemo session. I said hello and we hugged. She sat down and was telling me how she was doing when they called me back.

Dr. Steinberg came in and said, "you here again?" affectionately and sat down. I smiled and told him it was my last opportunity to ask him questions before I decided. I told him I was afraid and then I broke down crying. He said he understood. He told me again that his hope was that it wasn't in my bones and that had I not asked for the scan he would not have ordered it, but it was important for me to go through with it because I was experiencing pain.

He said that the pain is indicating that something is wrong and that oftentimes there are problems when there isn't any pain, so the fact that I am having it warrants investigation. He said that whatever my problems are, they are becoming uncomfortable and interfering in my life and one way or another we need to find out the cause. I told him about going to the chiropractor for my back pain and he said that once a person has had cancer, any pain they experience is observed for cancer related causes first, before any other treatment can be administered.

I told him part of the reason why I didn't want the scan is because I had already asked him what he would do if the cancer had spread and he told me I was already getting the most aggressive treatment. He responded by saying that what I am getting now is the most aggressive, standard therapy for my symptoms and diagnosis, but if my symptoms change, then he would use another approach. He said that there are other things they can do.

He told me that if there was cancer present in the bones, for example, it would have to be determined if any bone mass had been lost because there are drugs now available that actually build back bone mass. His point was that even if the results come back negative, there are other alternatives. He told me he knew I needed some hope to hold onto in the event this was the case.

I cried the whole time. I reminded him that I was going through this alone and he said he felt that was the hardest part for me. He told me that if it were his wife going through this, he would insist that she have the scan. He said that he didn't want me to "bury my head in the sand". I know he is right.

On a positive note, they tested my blood and again my counts are normal! I am happy about this. He reminded me that going through chemo was rough, physically and emotionally and I have been through five months of it. I told him I was tired of it and that I just wanted it to be over with and be healthy again. He assured me he would do everything in his power to achieve that.

I know my doctor is doing his best. I know that God is with me. It is up to me to keep holding onto the faith that I will get better and do everything I can to keep my spirits up and to stay positive and hopeful, no matter what happens from this point on.

November 4

Just got in from a grueling 8 hours in the classroom. I was the last to present my discussion and we ran out of time before I could do it. In a way I am relieved because it will give me more time to prepare and something else to focus on this upcoming week. I have another paper to write tomorrow and a debate to prepare for on Monday. Tonight I am not going to study. I am going to drink a glass of wine, light my candles, listen to my classical music, and relax.

November 5

I was in a tropical paradise. There were beautiful flowers all around me. It was warm and sunny and there was a beach with clear water and white sand. I took the kids and we went into the ocean. I kept finding money on the ground. Pretty soon I had an impressive stack of large bills.

We met my niece and she asked us to come and sleep over. When we got to her house, it was the old house I used to visit as a child (which is now a mental health center) and I was a little girl again. We walked in and someone was having a party. Members of the royal family were there and came up and spoke to me. I saw lots of people I knew and hadn't seen in a long time. We mingled for a while and then decided to go to bed. As we approached the stairs, I heard someone say, "Oh look, they live here in this mansion, what lucky girls".

As we walked up the stairs, I noticed my legs and feet and how perfect they were. I took the stairs, three and four at a time, watching my toes grab the carpet. She was amazed that I could climb the stairs this way. Then I realized the carpet was new. It once had been gold but it was a soft green, the color of healing. We got to the second floor and I walked into the bedroom and was admiring the sea of green carpet around me when I woke up.

Amazing: I talked to Dill on the phone today and he told me about a dream he had. In his dream, he was at a party and met a man who showed him the money in his wallet, which consisted of very large bills. At one point they climbed up a hill. The similarities in our dreams were uncanny and the fact that we had them the same night is unbelievable!

<u>November 6</u>

Yesterday was a pretty good day for me. I was in a good mood and was not worried. Every time I would think about the bone scan I would say to myself, "my bones are healthy". I imagined Dr. Steinberg saying, "Your scan was clear" over and over again. Not once did I allow any negative ideas into my head.

I went to sleep fairly well last night but woke up around 4 a.m. I did go back to sleep and got up again at 6:30. I showered and dressed and went to the imaging center at 8 a.m. The nuclear tech that did my muga scan is the same one who will do my bone scan. She gave me a shot and told me to come home and drink a lot of fluids and return at 10:45 for the test.

I asked her if she would see the results as she was scanning, or if it would be like an x-ray that had to be developed and she said she could see the results immediately but she could not tell me anything about it. I am nervous.

<u>Later:</u>

Went back to have the scan done. While the camera moved over me I repeated over and over in my head, "my bones are clear, my bones are clear". When it was over, I asked if I could look at the images without getting her opinion of the readings. Luanne showed them to me. I saw the bright white hot spots but there were a lot of them and they were symmetrical so I asked if some spots were normal. She said that where bones were close to the camera they would appear white.

She showed the image to the radiologist and he asked for four more pictures. She said that there was an area in my pelvis that he wanted to look at again. I saw the area she was talking about. It was directly between my hipbones on my spine. The areas I was concerned about did not seem abnormal to me. We finished up and I came home to study.

I went to class in a daze. I had a debate but wasn't really prepared. I got lucky because my professor decided we should discuss the issues briefly and then move on to the exam review. His previous class had debated for several hours on the same issue and he had to cut them short. He was tired and wanted to end class early. I was glad because my thoughts were elsewhere.

When I came home I got really down. I talked to Jim on the phone and he said that the kids were upset and worried about me. I began feeling remorse for the first time about breaking my family up. I wish I could take the pain away from my children and I can't.

<u>November 7</u>

I woke up to the phone ringing this morning around 8. It was Audrey from Dr. Steinberg's office. She said, "Hey lady, I just got your report and you are fine!" I said, "Oh my God, are you sure?" She laughed and said, "Yeah, let me read the fax," and she read it to me. I hung up the phone in tears. For about fifteen minutes I just sat there crying and saying, "Thank you God".

I made a few phone calls and then Jim brought the kids over. I am on cloud nine. I can finally see some light! The chemo and radiation can end this. I can be cured. I do have a chance to live a normal life again! I feel so relieved and thankful. The darkness that has been hanging over my head for the past month is finally disappearing.

<u>November 14</u>

Had chemo today and it went well. No messed up I.V.s, handled the Benadryl well, time went by fairly quickly, Dr. Steinberg was encouraging, CBC was excellent! It was a good visit.

Had my midterm in Growth and Development last night and made a 97. I am so glad! I have my project due Saturday and also another midterm so have been trying to study some. I also have to register for school that morning and Melanie the secretary told me to get there by 6 a.m. so I wouldn't have to stand in line. 6 a.m.!!! Usually the Saturday following chemo is a rough day for me with bone pains and I am a little concerned.

Since I got my bone scan results I really haven't thought much about "cancer". I have been keeping myself busy studying and spending good time with the kids and trying to just do my normal routine, cleaning house, paying bills, grocery shopping, running errands, etc. I have awakened every morning and immediately thanked God. My life has felt more normal in the past week than in several months now.

My little boy's birthday party was Saturday. He had a great time and I took lots of pictures. It was nice being around all the kids, doing the family thing. I cannot believe my baby is 8 years old. It just doesn't seem possible. I am so proud of him. He has handled all the changes in his life so very well. I make sure that when he talks, I listen.

I learned when he was little that if I wanted to find out what was bothering him, all I had to do was lie beside him at bedtime and just let him talk and eventually he would bring something up that was troubling him. I have been trying to do this more often now. He is strong, but sensitive. He communicates extremely well. He is an excellent student and has a 4.0 average in school. He likes nature and wants to be a field scientist. He loves music and telling jokes. His understanding of the world around him awes me. He is so mature for his age! When I look at him I just feel such overwhelming love for him. He is a beautiful child on the inside and the outside. He is so full of love and affection. We get along beautifully. He listens and obeys cheerfully and tried really hard to always do the "right thing". When we have difficulties, he talks to me and we communicate.

And my daughter, my little princess…is so beautiful, so charming. She is like a little butterfly, carefree and graceful, spreading her sunshine wherever she goes. She has always been "mommy's little girl". We have a very close bond. She needs so much affection! I hold her a lot and stroke her hair and kiss her and tell her how much I love her. She is creative and smart. She asks the most extraordinary questions! Her abstract thinking is highly developed, even at 5 years old! She is funny and sweet and she loves to laugh. I worry about her emotionally because she holds so much in. She very seldom cries. She tries to be so strong! She stepped on her brother's arm one night and hurt him and I could see she was upset so I went over and held her and watched her fight off tears for about 15 minutes.

What a blessing my children are! I absolutely cherish them. I am so thankful to God for allowing me to have such incredible kids. They amaze me. I am honored to be their mother. They are my best friends, my little buddies. I want so much for them! I want them to be happy. The times that I worry the most about having cancer are when I consider how tragic it would be for them if I died. I feel so helpless then. It breaks my heart. They are too young and innocent to have to go through all this!

I lie in bed at night and envision myself sharing the milestones in their lives…him graduating from high school and college, her getting married and having children…I try to see myself as an older woman full of life and joy and gratitude, looking on the positive side and being hopeful that I will continue to be here for them.

And I envision my own milestones…graduating with my Master's, working as a therapist, buying a house, and possibly getting married again one day. These are the things that keep me going, that give me hope.

<u>November 17</u>

I have spent the last few days with Bobbi and the children and we have enjoyed one another very much. It was wonderful having family around me. Last night I started hurting pretty bad and got worried about my class Saturday so today when it didn't seem any better I called my professor and talked to him about it. He is willing to work with me if I need more time to do my exam but I told him I would try to get through it. I have a long day ahead of me. The kids are spending the night with my mother so I don't have to wake them up to be at registration by 6 a.m. I am going to study for a while and try to get to sleep early tonight.

<u>November 18</u>

Got to school at 5:45 a.m. and registered for next term. I went to class, did my presentation, took my exam, then came home and went to sleep. Went to my mom's in the afternoon and cooked dinner and ate over there. I am tired.

<u>November 28</u>

Spent Thanksgiving week out of town. I had made the decision to either spend it with my sister Bobbi or with Dill, depending on how I felt. Since Jim was to keep the kids this week, I didn't want to be here. When I found out my blood counts were good, it was an easy decision. I drove up to New York on Tuesday morning. It took me 14 steady hours of driving in the freezing cold. I had to get out twice to refuel the car and thought I would freeze to death. When I finally got there, he was standing on the porch waiting for me. His mom drove up at the same time and we hugged. I went inside and he had a fuzzy comforter in the dryer and when I sat down he pulled it out and wrapped me up in it. I stayed at his mom's house and then later in the week we drove to Massachusetts and met his grandfather and other members of his family. We had thanksgiving dinner with his aunt and her family and although by this time I was really tired, I was happy to be there and enjoyed it. I saw mountains for the first time in my life…and a little snow too! The trip was hard on me but I didn't really feel bad the whole time, just weak. Being there felt so…comfortable. It was great to see him again. I had missed him so much! It was a nice trip and I was sad to leave.

The traffic was horrible on the way back down south and the drive took 16 hours!

I had an appointment at the cancer center today. My blood count was good but I was concerned about a large, hard mass under my incision. Dr. S told me to go see Dr. Pollard and have him look at it. While I was in the waiting room I felt some anxiety. He examined me, took out a needle, and drew out a lot of fluid. Afterwards, the knot was gone. I was so relieved! He laughed and said, "Don't worry, Betty, have faith in me". I said, "You have no idea how much faith I have in you!" I am to see him again in two weeks.

I missed the kids and couldn't wait to get them. I picked them up from school and they both rushed up to me and nearly jumped into my arms. We went out and bought a few items to decorate the apartment for Christmas and then stopped and bought meatball subs to bring home. I helped my son with his homework and we sat around talking for a while. It feels so good having them back with me again.

<u>December 2</u>

The past couple of nights I have slept extremely well. It is interesting to me that I no longer feel the pain in my legs or back like I did when I was worried about having the bone scan. I know without a doubt that mental attitude plays an important role in sickness and health. I do still have some discomfort in my abdomen but I wonder if maybe I have something like an ulcer. It certainly would make sense. When my mother was diagnosed with cancer 25 years ago I developed an ulcer. I was only 12 years old. I was treated and my symptoms gradually disappeared and I never really thought about it again until now. At some point, I want to look into this and try and find out the source of this discomfort.

I will only have health insurance coverage until Jim and I are divorced. Once I lose that policy I am sure I will no longer be able to get insurance. I can't help but wonder what I will do in the future. When I was trying to get government assistance it became clear to me how unfair the system is. If I had absolutely nothing and ten children with no husband, I would be getting a healthy check every month, but because I have a husband who supports his children, I am entitled to no financial help. It really pisses me off. I feel like I have worked long and hard enough in my life to support these programs and now that I need help there is none for me. I am thankful to be getting food stamps, but what happens if in the future I have to go through this again? I hope to have a job and a house one day soon…will I work hard to better my life and then lose it all again? It is so sad. I never understood how badly this country needs healthcare reform until now. If I lived in Canada, insurance would not be an issue.

Speaking of getting a house, I looked at another one today. This one was perfect. It was in a nice quiet subdivision on a back street with little traffic and backed up to a wooded area. It had a nice manicured lawn (and rose bushes!!) with a fenced-in back yard, perfect for the kids and my little Peanut the wiener-dog. There were lots of children playing throughout the neighborhood. The interior was well taken care of, with four bedrooms, two baths, and a beautiful great room with a high-beamed ceiling. It felt so right for me! The guy who owns it is willing to finance it for two and a half years until I can get financing on my own and the price is good for the market. He wants a small down payment that I could afford with no problem. The payments would be more than I am paying here but with an increase in child support from Jim (that he has already agreed to) I should be able to handle it. I want this house so badly!

What a difference having a house like this would make in the kids' lives! They would have a yard to play in again, their own rooms like they are accustomed to, and even a playroom. They could have their friends over to spend the night like before and even have birthday parties at home if they wanted. The house is about a mile from their school and about two miles from the place where I am hoping to start working. Not only that, but it is just blocks from my niece's apartment and about a half mile from my mother and brother. I just keep telling myself that if it is meant for me, I will get it.

There is another woman who has made an offer on it and was to let the owner know today if she was going to sign the contract so I will just have to wait and see what happens. It is a huge decision for me to make during a very uncertain time in my life but I just feel like it would be such a positive change of environment for all of us that the commitment would be negligible.

After I looked at the house I picked up the kids from school and came home and started dinner. Jim came over to bring me our artificial Christmas tree and part of the decorations. He said that when he pulled the boxes out of the attic he remembered that last year the tree was still up in the house when I left and he got really emotional. I hugged him for the first time in a year. I was cooking chicken and he laughed and said that the thing he missed the most about me was my fried chicken. I asked him if he wanted to eat dinner with us but he said no.

The children had a blast putting up the tree. I let them do everything except the lights. They are so excited about Christmas. I loved Christmas when I was a child. I would sit by the tree and just stare at it all night. It was so beautiful and magical. I sat down on the sofa while they were hanging the ornaments and smiled. I am so thankful that I am alive and able to share this with them!

<u>December 5</u>

Tonight I sent this letter out to all my friends and family:

Hello all

Just an update...today I had my last chemo treatment: five hours with an I.V., four medications, blood work and lab work, all while watching TV and talking with my sister Bobbi and the other patients I have gotten to know from going to the cancer center. I got lots of hugs from the staff (they are so wonderful). Dr. Steinberg, my oncologist, congratulated me on suffering through five long months of treatment and doing a great job that he was proud of. I hope none of you ever have to go through this but if you ever do, Dr. Steinberg is the best! They pinned me with a button that said, "I Graduated From Chemotherapy" :)

Although this marks a major milestone in my treatment, it is far from over. I am having some problems associated with lymphedema, which is a condition caused by the removal of the axillary lymph nodes. Since they are gone, the lymphatic fluid builds up in a pocket under my arm and has to be drained with a needle periodically. In two weeks I will start daily radiation, which will last for six weeks. I will begin taking Tamoxifen, an anti-cancer drug and will continue on this for five years. During that time I will be constantly monitored for cancer. I am happy to be this far along and looking forward to having some semblance of a normal life the beginning of next year.

The week I was diagnosed with breast cancer I was also hired at the insurance company but couldn't accept the job because of the uncertainty of the treatment. It is my plan to begin working there as soon as my radiation is complete in February.

As you may know, I have been looking for a place to move because my lease here expires Feb. 1. Last Friday I found a beautiful house and put a deposit on it. It has tenants in place until Dec. 15 and then after Christmas I can begin moving. I am thrilled about having more room, a yard, and a neighborhood again for the kids. They have been my little prayer warriors through all this...I am so thankful to have such wonderful children.

In two weeks I will be finished with my first term of graduate school. So far it is going well, although I have had a difficult time focusing on my work. I am in the midst of writing a research paper on Divorce and so am looking forward to getting it done and finishing up the term.

I want to thank all of you for your concern and prayers. You helped fill many lonely and desperate hours for me and I love you all very much for it!

When I get settled into the house, I hope to have lots of company, so consider this an open invitation to visit!

Thanks again and please continue to remember me, Jim, and the children in your prayers.

Love, peace and health...
Betty Henson

Today after chemo Bobbi and I went out for lunch and she treated me. I was really hungry and ate everything on my plate! Afterwards, we stopped by our mother's and said hello. Then I drove Bobbi by the house to look at it. She was so excited for us!

I haven't yet told the kids about the house because I know they will be anxious to see it and I don't feel comfortable going over there while the tenants are still living there, especially since they are busy with moving.

We went and picked the kids up from school and were to stop by the grocery store on the way back. As I got out of the car to go in, I was hit with stomach cramps and nausea and had to forego grocery shopping and come home. Bobbi left to go to her vacation house locally where her husband is staying this week.

I had diarrhea by this time and lay down on the sofa and ended up taking a very long nap, with no interruptions from the kids! I could hardly believe it. They played quietly in their bedroom for at least two hours and when I woke up I was in a good mood and felt much better, aside from the stomach upset.

I am to go back to the cancer center for my CBC workup next Tuesday and Friday and then that should be all my contact with them until I finish my radiation. I would like to do something nice for the staff and Dr. Steinberg to thank them. I enjoyed getting to know them all and want to express my appreciation.

Today when I saw Dr. Steinberg I told him that five years ago I went to another doctor about a swollen lump under my ribcage that she said was a lymph gland. I wanted him to check it for me since this was my last regular visit. He laughed and said, "You don't have any lymph nodes there!" I said, "I don't? Then what is it?" He told me it was a fat globule and I laughed and said, "What do I do about a swollen fat globule? Wait, I know, lose weight, right?" He got a good laugh off that one and commented that my previous doctor should go back to med school and retake her anatomy classes...scary.

I told my landlord that I bought a house and he wants me to prepare a written termination. I have to pay my rent tomorrow and will take this over then. I know I have a lot of work ahead of me that will be difficult but I am very excited over the changes taking place in my life!

<u>December 6</u>

I didn't sleep at all last night! I really don't know why except I was thinking about Dill. He has been busy with schoolwork for the past few days and I have not talked to him for more than just a few minutes at a time since I got back from visiting him. I guess I just miss him. I watched that clock hour to hour until I finally had to get up at 7:00 and get the kids off to school. I drove by the house on the way home…it is so nice! I can't wait to move!

I came home and got started on the telephone. I had lots of calls to make. I was on the phone until about noon and then lay down to take a nap. I woke up around 3 p.m. and got dressed, went to the bank, then the grocery store, then picked the kids up from school.

We came home and made sausage dogs and chili (which I could not have eaten a few weeks ago), ate dinner, and watched TV. I got them ready for bed and worked on my research paper for a while, then caught up on my email. I had lots of letters from people encouraging me and congratulating me on finishing up chemo. My friend in Greece wrote that she was so impressed with all the changes in my life and how I was handling them. She said she never knew what a "tough cookie" I was, but then I "never had to be before". She is so right.

Bobbi called me and said that I sounded great. She said my voice was full of energy and enthusiasm. This was nice to hear. Although I feel pretty tired and not energetic, I know that my attitude has improved a great deal this week.

Tomorrow I am to have a telephone consultation with my attorney so that I can get my settlement money to close on the house. I also have to interview a local counselor here for a paper I am doing in my therapeutic counseling class. I am to meet with my study group at noon to write the abstract for our research paper and then am to meet Joe (the owner of the house) to pick up some papers from him. Bobbi is to meet me back here by 2 p.m. and will go with me to pick up the kids and then she is spending the night with me tomorrow night and Friday night. I will have class all day Saturday. Busy, busy, busy.

December 10

Well, am on the downside of pain now. My last side effects from the last chemo.

I went to class yesterday and it was a great experience. One of my fellow students did a class presentation on alternative forms of therapy. She brought in an African drum and several water bottles and we pounded rhythmically until the whole class was in unison. It was such a stress reliever! And fun!

I got my midterm exam back and made an A. I also made an A on my class presentation. I am really happy about this, considering I did both on a day when I was in a lot of pain and exhausted from not sleeping the night before. I am confident now in my ability to successfully complete graduate school.

The past few days I have been in a mild depressed state. I hesitate to call it that because it sounds so negative. I feel like I have been living in semi-dream state since I found out I had breast cancer. It is like the whole world became less real and I began looking through a fog of uncertainty. I know that it is my pattern to escape from reality and I believe that is what I have done for several months.

Now that I am being forced to move forward, beyond chemo, I am hoping to see things with more clarity. I know that the decision to divorce my husband is one that has negatively impacted my children and my family relationships. I know that I have subjected myself to living alone without the security of a companion to be there with me during rough times ahead. I think about this constantly.

One thing I have become aware of as a result of this past year is how weak I was in relationships. I was always willing to do what would make others happy and ignore my own desires. I expected to receive back as much as I gave and when I didn't get it, felt resentment because of it. Am I ready to move into an intimate relationship with someone else?

I believe that the more we learn about ourselves, the better we are able to connect with others. It is so hard, looking at who you are, with all your faults. It is painful.

December 20

Sent this letter out today:

Hello All!

Just an update here...started radiation therapy this week. I was fascinated. Two techs painted colored lines all over my chest and side to guide the lasers...and I might add that I am ticklish so this was not pleasant although I giggled throughout the three hours it took to create this masterpiece. The curiosity got to me and I couldn't wait until the end to see this work of art; lifted my head to look at it and smeared bright red permanent ink all underneath my chin...you should see the stares I get :P

I am not being treated with Cobalt but rapidly fired, guided electrons instead. They pass over me and intersect at targets painted on my body. Did you know that a physician can maneuver your body in such a way that he can feel both lobes of your liver with his hands? Me neither until this week...not very comfortable, but I thought it was interesting ☺.

*On the home front, I am hoping to move into a new home by the end of the year. I will be doing a lease option and will have the choice of buying this house in a couple of years. *crosses fingers**

In about 8 weeks I can begin working again...YAY! I finally got hired for the position I have been wanting and will most likely take that job but am considering possibly looking for something in my field before I make the final decision. I will have to do an internship in a mental health facility at the end of this year so it would be helpful to have a job in place already.

I just finished my first term of school....wow....what a learning experience. If you want to know more about yourself, take a graduate course in therapeutic counseling, hahaha. I am proud to report that I pulled a 4.0 while going through chemo...probably the biggest accomplishment of my life, next to giving birth :)

I am feeling pretty good considering all that has transpired over the past six months. I am tired of course, and I know I have a long road ahead but I am so very thankful the worst part of treatment is over. Not only that, but my hair is beginning to come back...it's only a faint shadow, but nonetheless, IT'S HAIR! (I will miss not having to shave my legs, however, hahaha)

*Thanks again to all of you for your encouragement, visits, phone calls, letters, etc. Don't know how I would have made it without the support of people around me *big hug**

"That's how love works, that's how love moves, like a river running through you...Sometimes it lifts you as high as Heaven, it consumes you, but that's a given...
That's how love moves" - Faith Hill

Love to all and have a blessed Christmas!
Betty Henson

December 27

Christmas is over. It was nice but I am glad. On the 22nd my mother went into the hospital with chest pains. I had dropped the children off at her house that morning so I could go sign the contract on the house I found. She called Jim to come get the kids and he took her to the emergency room. I got there around 5 p.m. and he left so the kids and I stayed at the hospital until about 7:30 p.m. until I knew that she was stable. They admitted her and we were afraid that she would be there through Christmas but they determined it was not her heart and let her come home on Christmas Eve. They believe her chest pains were caused by an area of her lungs that look suspicious on x-ray and could be related to her emphysema or cancer. They don't know yet. You know, it's funny but my dad died on December 14 and every year since then my mother has gotten sick. This makes the sixth time. I think the stress of the holidays is too much for her to take without him. I wonder how much of this could be avoided.

I ended up buying all the food for dinner with my food stamps and cooked the meal that my mother was going to. It turned out really good. We spent the night at her house so Santa could visit there. I was worried that the children would be disappointed with Christmas because it was so lean compared to previous years but they didn't notice at all.

I enjoyed the time I spent with my family. There didn't seem to be any tension and things went smoothly. Jim came and got the kids and then I spent that night over there too to clean up the mess. The next day I didn't wake up until after 2:30 p.m.! Guess I was tired! I went and paid the deposit to have my electricity turned on at the house and came home.

I had a long talk with Jim on the phone. In the past week the kids have talked a lot about "Daddy's friend Laura". Evidently this is a woman he has been spending a good bit of time with. She has been out with them to dinner and visited at the house and the kids both think she is nice.

The night of Jim's company Christmas party I had the children and he wanted me to get them dressed nicely so they could go with him. When he came to pick them up, I asked him if Laura was going and he admitted she was. This angered me that he would have the nerve to ask me to dress up my children so he could take them on a date while we are still legally married and worse, of all places, to his company party. We communicated pretty well and I believe he understood my concerns and promised to leave the children out of his relationship until we are divorced.

I have such mixed feelings about all this. I realize I am afraid to let go of Jim. I know that things could have been a lot better in our marriage but they also could have been a lot worse. I devoted the best 15 years of my life to him. I was young and healthy and attractive when we got married. I feel like I've thrown all those years away. It scares me to think about being alone in the future now that I have had cancer. Not only that, but it makes me sad to see him accomplishing things that I knew he would and assumed I would be part of. I hurt for the children too. But I know also that all these reasons are not reasons for staying in a relationship. It has to be for love…not for convenience or security. And when I think about the times that I was sick and alone and he was so mean to me it makes me realize that I am better off without him.

Still, I wonder if things would have been better if I would have tried harder. I thought that by the end of our year's separation the answers would be clearer to me but it is just as much a fog as it was then. When it comes to relationships, nothing makes sense. If I consider my life without complicating it with thoughts of what "could be" then I know I am doing what is best. Given the choices I have, I think I am doing the right thing. If I end up alone, then I end up alone but I will have arrived at that point without being a victim, but rather, acting on my own power to achieve the most I could, independent of others.

I think about Dill all the time and wish that he were closer so we could spend more time together. One night on the phone I all but begged him to move down here right away and immediately afterwards I regretted it. As badly as I want that, I know that I have to allow him to decide on his own what he wants to do and make the effort to act on it. I cannot allow myself to push him. I have to let him do it.

It would be great to have him in my life, even though I worry a little about my ability to sustain a "new" relationship. I guess I don't feel like I have as much to offer as I did before I had cancer. I certainly look much worse, feel bad, have no energy, and have a very uncertain future. I have debts and bills and soon will not have insurance. I believe that may have a lot to do with my new ambiguity about the divorce.

I hope as the days go by and I begin to feel better this will all change. The one thing that is clear to me is that I have to focus less on others and more on myself. This is the time to take care of me. I am trying to just let things happen the way they are meant to be. I cannot control the future so I just have to let go and trust that it will all work out for the best.

February 7, 2001

Well it has been quite a while since my last entry. So much has happened! Up until just a few days ago, my fingertips were still numb from Chemo. I started my radiation 6 weeks ago. It was really difficult making the effort to be there every single day, but I am down to my last 5 treatments and am hanging in there. The most discomfort I have experienced has been in just the last couple of weeks. I am burned visibly and my skin is peeling off in places. It itches like crazy but I cannot scratch or use ointment because it causes my target lines to rub off. The people at the radiation clinic are very nice. It is a humbling experience but I am doing well.

Today Dill got his degree in the mail. I was so happy for him and proud of his accomplishment. I believe he is planning to work for a while and save up some money and then possibly try to move down south. I want this so badly! It has been hard not having the companionship of the person I care about so deeply. I get very lonely sometimes. At these times, it upsets me that Jim has someone in his life on a regular basis. It makes me jealous. I had words with him today over just that and then I realized later that it may be displaced anger over my frustration with Dill being so far away.

I am still in school, working on my second term in the counseling program. So far I have an A average. I had to miss one class last week because my mother was in the ICU unit at the hospital and the doctors were unsure as to whether she would make it through the night. I sat in her room and watched her heart rate, respiration and oxygen saturation drop to zero 8 times. I was terrified that she would die each time and I watched her, waiting for her chest to stop moving and her eyes to glaze over like my father's did when he died. It was horrible. Fortunately she has improved a great deal and on my visit with her today her spirits were good and I felt relieved.

I moved into my "new" house on January 1. I love it and so do the children. It is a small house but it has four bedrooms (one is my computer room) and a nice fenced-in back yard. The neighborhood is great...there are so many children! For the first time in their lives, the kids are able to ride their bikes in the street without worrying about cars speeding by. I feel safe here. I feel like I am home.

The medical bills are pouring in. I am getting collection letters with nasty little handwritten notes on them. It makes me feel terrible but there is nothing I can do. Jim has been good over the past few months advancing me money out of my divorce settlement so I can pay my bills. I am thankful for that.

As of January 28, we were separated for a year. As soon as our paperwork is finished, we can divorce.

February 14

Today I had my last radiation treatment. I am so glad this is over. I learned a lot about myself throughout my cancer treatment. I believe I am a much more genuine person now. I have grown up a lot. I am learning to be my own friend.

The techs asked me today how I was going to celebrate. I told them I was going to go home and have a 24 hour date with my bed with no interruptions. I am just so tired.

I came very close to tears as I was leaving the clinic, and again when I got home. Today is Valentine's Day and once again, I am alone. I plan to make some popcorn and watch T.V.

Tomorrow I get the children back, thank heaven. I miss them so much.

March 6

I'm sitting here in the computer room with the kids and the pets. My son is bugging me to play one of his computer games, my daughter is reading out of her book, and the dog and cat are wrestling on the floor.

I enjoy my kids so much. They are the light of my life. Tonight they talked a lot about Jim's girlfriend Laura. It started to get on my nerves but I held my composure. I finally sat them down and told them that I thought it was okay for Daddy to be having a friend spend time with him and it was alright with me for them to like her. They talked a little about her and then changed the subject.

Last night was my final for class. I will start again in about 10 days. I think I did well but will have to wait and see.

My skin is healing well and I am beginning to get some feeling back under my arm and on my shoulder. My scars aren't as horrible looking now. I guess I am just getting used to seeing them.

March 23

I am sitting here drinking my morning coffee and trying to get up the energy to clean house. For the past few weeks I have suffered incredible fatigue. I have learned that this is called CRF (Cancer Related Fatigue) and is a legitimate and serious concern for cancer patients. It is unlike anything I have ever experienced. I get up and walk to the mailbox and get winded. I clean house for 15 minutes and have to sit down for 20. I go to bed at night and wake up the next day as tired as I was when I went to bed. It is hard to imagine working full time again feeling this way.

Two weeks ago I went to the temporary staffing office where I used to work and asked them to place me again. I worked one day in an interior decorator's office. I went in at 8:30 and by noon I was exhausted and wondering how I could possibly make it until 5. I ate a light lunch and rested my back, got a second wind and managed to stick it out until almost 4:00 pm. I was happy I was able to do it.

The next week I worked three days straight. I was sitting down the whole time and didn't have any problems. It was wonderful to just dress up and go to work as if things were normal again. I didn't talk about cancer and as far as I know the people I was working with had no idea. I wore my wig of course because my hair is so short. I have just begun in the past few days to brave going outside and in public without it. It feels odd and I am self-conscious but am glad that it is finally growing back some.

Jim and I are getting along pretty well. He asked me last weekend if I wanted to go skating with him and the kids and of course I did. I didn't want to miss being with them. I put on skates and, remembering how much I used to love skating when I was a child, hopped up and took off and immediately fell down and busted my butt! He didn't even offer to help me up and I was in pain. I hurt my back and bruised my hand, elbow, and hip. The next morning I felt like I had been in a car wreck! My wrist was purple. I had tried to break my fall and had landed with all my weight on that side. For a couple of days I thought it was broken. Melanie (the secretary at school) called to see why I wasn't in class because she was worried about me. I ended up having to drop one of my classes since I missed the first day. This will put my graduation date off by a few weeks but there was just no way I could go.

Jim promised me a while back that he would keep his girlfriend away from the kids until we were divorced but he hasn't done it. Quite the opposite has happened. My daughter draws pictures of herself holding hands with Laura and writes "I love you" on the pictures. She even asked me if I would mail one to Laura for her! I was shocked but I tried not to let it show. She wears a bracelet that Laura gave her for her birthday and it is obvious how much she likes her. I hope this woman realizes how much she has affected my little girl. If that relationship doesn't work out, she is going to be hurt. It makes my blood boil just to think about it. On top of all that, it is embarrassing to me that people I know have seen them all out together while we are still married and I am sick. He is not trying to hide it at all. I talked with him about this and told him that I would have preferred we both keep our relationships private from the children until the divorce but since he was so open about his, I had no intention of continuing to hide my relationship with Dill any longer.

On the evening of Valentine's Day I was somewhat down. After getting cards and flowers every Valentine's Day for 15 years, it has been hard to not get anything the past two years. I sat down that night at the computer and had a "virtual bouquet" of roses from Dill. I cried when I saw it. Then later that night, he called and gave me news that made my day. He said that he had decided to set a goal by April 15 to tell me when he was moving down here. Again, I cried. So the decision has been made. It is no longer an "if" but now a "when". He is working hard to try and make enough money to make the move. I am so excited!

I told Jim that Dill had decided to move down sometime this year. He said, "Oh boy" with a look of disgust on his face and "Now I guess I will know what it's like to hear the kids constantly talk about the new person in your life". In a way it felt good to see him consider the hurt I have been going through. I think if Dill were down here already it wouldn't bother me to hear them talk about his girlfriend. I really don't have anything against her. I know she has no children and doesn't understand the love and concern I have for the emotional welfare of my children and how she could be jeopardizing that. I blame my ex-husband for being irresponsible with her, but what is done is done. They seem to be getting along well and I hope this continues. I look forward to the day when they can meet Dill too and we can all spend time together as well. He seems excited too to meet them and I am so grateful for this.

I went to see Dr. Steinberg Wednesday for my follow up exam. They drew blood and told me they would test me for cancer markers (proteins in the blood that may suggest a tumor) and elevated liver function (enzymes in the blood that may suggest damage to the liver). He examined my breasts and lymph nodes and said everything felt good and he was pleased with my progress. He said my color was good and I looked great. I asked him if he had ever consider hiring a counselor to work with his patients and he said he had in fact given it some thought. I told him that when I got licensed I would come back and ask him for a job. We talked a little about that and then I left.

When I was at the checkout desk, some of the staff I knew came up to hug me and chat. They asked me how Dill was doing and I blushed a little and smiled. They were teasing me, saying "Look! She's in love!". It was cute and sweet and made me feel good. It is true that when I talk about him my whole face just lights up. My sister has told me the same. When things get to be too much for me, I can think about him and feel good. I need that now. I doubt it will last but for right now, it is a good thing.

My mother has been in and out of the hospital since Christmas. Her blood sugar is erratic and last week she suffered a stroke that left her paralyzed on the left side. She is so pitiful it breaks my heart to see her. The doctors are sending her to a nursing home next Monday. Sometimes I think about not having parents and I get really sad. I always thought my mom and dad would be there for me if I ever needed them but it hasn't turned out that way. At this time in my life when I really need my family, I have no one but Bobbi I can count on…but at least I have her. She has been wonderful to me and continues to be my biggest ally. I am still hoping she will move back home but that remains to be seen.

I am still trying to just live in the present and enjoy myself as much as I can. It has been a lot of fun playing with my kids and their neighborhood friends. I am enjoying my classes and am excited about going back to work full time. I am hoping to interview next week for the position I have been waiting for since last June. I may be able to finalize the divorce as early as next week. There are a lot of things going on and I can see my life taking shape again. I thank God for every day that I feel good enough to get out of bed and get dressed and I am hopeful that this disease is a thing of the past for me.

The one thing I am certain of is that I am a fighter. If I didn't know this before, I do now. I am proud of myself for the way I have handled the obstacles in my life this past year and I feel stronger than ever.

March 22, 2002

I have avoided this diary for quite some time now. A year in fact. So much has changed. My mother died in April last year. She had a stroke and had to be placed into a nursing home. She really hated it and never got over it. The last time I saw her, I went to visit at the home and took her for a walk in a wheelchair around the grounds. We had a nice visit and she kept telling me to do what makes me happy and that I was strong and I would find what I was looking for one day. I miss her.

My half-brother and half-sister were cruel to me after Mama's death. I don't want to go into the tedious details. Let me just suffice to say that they made some decisions that I didn't agree with and couldn't understand. Some things were said that were hurtful and no one offered apologies. We became even more estranged than before. I think the hardest issue in my life so far has been to try and forgive them for hurting me so badly. Every time I think about it my heart aches. I feel like I did what I could to try and address the problems but in the end I realized that I was wasting my time. I really wanted them to be different people and it wasn't possible. They expressed that they did not want me in their lives and so I had to gradually accept it and move on.

I ended up writing in detail about the oddities of my family for a class I took in Family Systems. I shared the family history and constructed a genogram, showing all the broken relationships in the family. It was quite revealing. My professor told me that it was the best analysis and counseling proposal he had seen in many years of teaching that class. I realized then that I did have an understanding of the problems in the family and that I wasn't necessarily the dysfunctional member even though they tried to make me feel that way. It was refreshing to have someone on my side for a change.

My ex-husband has decided now to marry his girlfriend. I think it is significant that they are planning their wedding for January 1, the same date as when I left him. I wonder if she realizes her anniversary will be on the same day as the anniversary of our separation.

I have talked with her on the phone a couple of times but I have not yet met her. Last year around August I had a depressive episode the week prior to what would have been my tenth wedding anniversary. I was struggling to make some meaning out of everything that had happened in my marriage and made the mistake of calling my ex and asking him to talk to me, to help me. He was uppity and cold and I regretted calling him. Since then, I have tried to accept the circumstances but have made it very clear to him that I feel like he should have been more supportive of me regardless of our separation during the time I was so sick.

I wish that people could be more real. If you are angry, say so. If I have insulted you, tell me. I think if we were all more honest and open with our feelings, we would all be a lot happier. I am so tired of the mind games that people play because they don't want to reveal their true feelings.

A couple of weeks ago I visited Dr. Steinberg for my checkup. It has been almost two years since I was diagnosed. So far I am clean and I thank God for that. It has been a rough recovery. I still do not have feeling in my shoulder or breast. I can tell the radiation damaged my heart. I also have not yet recovered from the cancer related fatigue. My energy level is much better these last couple of months than it has been since all this started but of course I am not back to my old self.

About Dill. He moved to S.C. last May. I was so happy! My expectations of our relationship were unrealistic though…I expected it to be like a marriage…but we hadn't even dated yet. Things were strained for a while. I have so much admiration for him to do what he did because he didn't know what he was getting into. A new girlfriend with my medical issues, children, a new state…total culture shock. But he coped with the challenges well. I cannot say it was easy because it wasn't. He was used to being alone and I was used to being codependent. He had a hard time finding a job and even when he did, the pay down here is so much lower than up North that money has been non-existent for him. This put a damper of course on our relationship because neither one of us had money to go out or do much of anything.

There was a while when I was very frustrated at this point, ready to move forward faster. I guess when you have had cancer, you don't want to waste any time. I felt like it was obvious that I "should" be on the fast track and that he "should" be too. Lately we have had quite a few "discussions" about this. Would I like to get married to him?

Yes. But I am finding out that I can live alone and be content. I am enjoying my house and my responsibilities and finally feeling like I can carve out a life for myself, with or without another.

I think I have grown up since last year. I have decided that the most important things in my life now are my children and learning to love myself. My career is driving me now. I did get a job and met some great people. I worked there for about a month when I was offered a counseling job at an agency in Conway. I was so thrilled!

The money was great, the benefits, retirement....I went to work full of energy and enthusiasm and was doing a good job I think until my supervisor started flirting with me. I couldn't believe what was happening. When it got to the point where he demanded that it be me to go out of town with him at the last minute, I reported him to the administration and it was downhill from there. I expected them to be ethical and do an investigation. I was wrong. I lasted three months at that job before they fired me. It was the first time in my life I had been fired from a job. They said it was due to a reduction in force because of budgetary constraints but I know otherwise. I squealed and they shut me up. It was a lesson well taken.

I am back on food stamps and Medicaid again. I am living off child support and student loans. I am due to start my counseling internship next week and so I am going to try and pay my bills as best I can until I graduate and then look for work again. I can't believe I am almost finished with school! I still have an A average which I am very proud of. I have also decided that it is time for me to make my own mark on society and I have become involved in some organizations that I feel will benefit me professionally.

Tonight for example I am on call at the Rape Crisis Center. I am a victim's advocate. I will also be working with the abuse shelter soon. I have joined the Literacy Council and have been invited to become a member of a local organization. Meanwhile, I am trying to come to terms with life as a single woman. Period. No future expectation of marriage or family. Just me and the kids, trying to keep the demons at bay. I know I am in for a lonely ride but I need this. I need to be able to depend upon myself for the first time in my life. I need to be successful taking care of me. Being a good mother, a good student, a good community servant, and eventually a good counselor...those are my goals now.

June 28

Sitting here looking at my reflection on the monitor. My hair is down to my shoulders now. It's curlier than before. It began growing back white and I shaved it, then it grew back ashy gray. Finally the brown started coming back in. One day I was driving my car with the sunroof open, looked in the rear view mirror and shouted, Oh my gosh, my hair has red highlights again! I was so happy. The hair thing is good now. I love it.

Dill's mom gave me an annual state park pass for my birthday and the kids and Dill and I have gone to the beach quite a lot. We all have suntans now.

I have gained about twenty pounds since I started chemo. I eat anything I want now and I have the energy to go all day and do basically whatever I want but then when I get home I do get tired and I have definitely gotten good use out of my couch in the past year.

Things have really come around for me. This is my last month of school. I will get my masters in about 5 weeks. I am extremely proud of myself. I still love my house and have managed to never be late on a payment...amazing considering I haven't had a steady job in over five years.

I recently was hired by an alcohol and drug abuse agency and was supposed to start work Monday but found out last week I have to have a hysterectomy. Dr. Pierce is concerned that the combination of my erratic periods and the daily doses of Tamoxifen I am taking will cause me to develop cancer in my uterus so we are eliminating that risk. The director of the agency graciously agreed to let me wait and start my job in August. I can't wait to start working again. I know this surgery will be rough but I can do it.

Dill and I have had some real ups and downs since he moved down here, but now that it has settled down a little it's really nice. Our relationship has taught me a great deal about myself. I am learning to love myself and see myself as a whole, complete being. That was his goal from the beginning, was to help me with that issue. I am learning to respect myself and my independence and self-sufficiency. I recently received a scholarship from the American Business Women's Association. They have invited me to join their organization. I would like to do this. I have also received awesome recommendation letters from my professors and my resume is really taking shape. I am considering applying to a university in Florida that has an online doctoral program. Why not?

<u>September 6</u>

This is the entry I had hoped I would never have to write. The cancer has come raging back.

I breezed through my hysterectomy and recovered extremely rapidly. Four weeks later I started my new job. I cannot express how happy that job made me. The people there are absolutely wonderful. They were so loving and accepting of me.

I threw myself into working again for the first time in…how long now? I can't even remember when things seemed normal. I had to drive 40 minutes to work and back every day and two days a week I was working 12 hour shifts because I was doing group therapy in the evenings.

I was getting into the groove of things, feeling more competent about my duties and my physical ability to handle work again when I began to feel bad. Headaches.

When I first noticed it, I thought it was just from fatigue and my back hurting. Then I began to run a fever and thought maybe it was sinuses. But the sinus medicine didn't help. Finally I went to the chiropractor for an adjustment and for a couple of days I felt better.

One day I was driving home from work and I noticed my vision was blurry. I began to get light headed and dizzy and I got scared. I called Dill on my car phone and told him. I just needed him to talk to me as I drove so I could make it. The feeling passed fairly quickly and I got home but I knew something was terribly wrong.

What if it was Brain Cancer? My most feared. It was the one that I used to skip over when I was reading about Breast Cancer Metastasis. It was the one I was most afraid of. Daddy always told me that my knowledge was the one thing that no one would ever be able to take away from me and so I guess I always coveted my intelligence. The thought of one day losing my mind and all it's functioning was too much to bear.

I made friends with a fellow counselor at the agency and he saw how much pain I was in day in and day out. He came into my office and asked me why I was being so stubborn about not going to the doctor and so in a weak moment I confided in him about having had cancer. He told me I should go right away. I knew he was right. I left work right then and went to the emergency room.

Of course they didn't find anything. I was hoping for a sinus infection or West Nile Virus…herniated discs….anything…..but they found nothing….X-rays clean. Next stop, MRI. I knew what to do. I stoically called Dr. Steinberg and told him I needed an MRI. I wanted to have it done before I saw him. He ordered it for the next morning.

I drifted through the procedure like always, not really thinking about cancer. I had two hours before my appointment to get the results but I couldn't go home and come back. I went to the cancer center and waited in the car. When I finally went inside, the nurses that I knew came out to say hello and hug me. They were too friendly. I was nervous.

The rest is like a blur. I remember hearing myself explain my symptoms, as if there was any other reason for them, like I was trying to convince the doctor. He leaned against the counter and looked compassionately at me and just let me go on. Eventually my voice trailed off. I could see it in his eyes. He said they found spots on the MRI in my brain…12 to 15 of them that they could see clearly enough to count but there was probably more. There was no surgery and chemo wouldn't cross the blood brain barrier…there is not enough blood vessels in the brain to deliver the chemo to the tumors. The only treatment would be whole head radiation, which could leave me permanently bald and/or impaired mentally but may only add a couple of months to my life. My prognosis? 2 months.

<u>October 22, 2003</u>

Well. It's been over a year now and I'm still here! After Dr. S. told me the bad news, I went to work as quickly as I could. I had a conference with my supervisor and the director of the agency and they hugged me, cried and prayed for me. I told them that because I could not longer drive, I'd have to give up my position right away. This broke my heart because I loved my job. My director insisted that I not clean out my office and not resign. He offered to continue to pay me as long as he could. I was so grateful for that. I said my goodbyes to everyone and left. In one week's time, I planned my funeral, asked my former boss and friend who was a pastor to deliver my eulogy, wrote my obituary, wrote my will, power of attorney, health care proxy, and that's not all.
I wrote my wedding vows too!

When I told Dill my news, he asked me to marry him! I was thrilled but of course wish it had been different circumstances. I started planning a wedding and when I told my best friend in Greece, she insisted that we come to visit her in on our honeymoon. On September 14, 2002 my sister Bobbi married us while we were barefoot in the ocean in front of castle ruins at our State Park. The kids were there and made the prettiest, most photogenic pictures I've ever seen of them. We went to an exclusive restaurant to have dinner and wedding cake afterwards and then we had a honeymoon in Greece. Greece was awesome…following are excerpts from the journal I kept of our trip.

<u>October 2</u>

My Internship Supervisor gave me this gorgeous little journal. She came to visit just after Dill and I had planted Chrysanthemums along the sidewalk. It had been a good day for me. I promised her I would carry this journal to Greece and that is exactly what I am doing!

My writing is not very good because we are flying over the Atlantic Ocean at 37,000 ft. in turbulence! I think we are about halfway between Nova Scotia and the UK but it has been awhile since the last update. I am on the aisle and my husband Dill (I just love saying that!) is sitting by the window asleep. We have been in the air now for about 5 hours. I asked for vegan meals and so when they brought my dinner it was fruit, a radish salad, couscous with beans, a veggie patty, rice, and steamed broccoli and carrots. It was really good…I have been juicing for so long that it was nice to have a full meal for a change.

It's hard to believe last night we were at Pat's house in the hot tub! On the way to NY, I mentioned to Dill that I had never been to the Capitol so he gave me a tour! Now I can say I've seen the squirrels on the White House lawn!

Dill teased me because when we started out that morning I didn't realize how long it had been since I tweezed my eyebrows and in the morning sun it was yuk! So I started with the eyebrows, which led to other things and before I knew it I had spent 14 hours in 2 increments: doing my face and sleeping!

My mother-in-law's friend drove us to JFK and we parked ourselves in a lounge overlooking the runways. We started talking to a cute Polish girl and her friend. It turns out that she made more money working in a month in an amusement park in the US than her mother makes in a year in Poland!

Well, this big bird is shaking pretty hard now and I am having a lot of trouble writing. I think I will try to make my way to the "water closet" and the see if I can round up a cup of tea.

Later

The turbulence has calmed down and we are flying over Dublin, Ireland. It is nighttime now and all the streetlights are on below. It reminds me of spider webs, only golden and sparkling. It is beautiful. It didn't take very long to arrive in Frankfurt, Germany where we had a lengthy layover. We drank espresso in a very modern glass and chrome café and then went to an observation area where we watched the sunrise. I lay down across a row of seats and finally fell asleep.

When it was time to board the plane, I busted my butt in front of so many people…It was hysterical and humiliating at the same time. We were on this long conveyor belt taking us to our gate when I notice my water bottle that was on top of my carry-on (ya know the piece of luggage that has your passports and all your important stuff in it) was empty!

I panicked and squatted to remove all the wet papers and was trying to salvage them when the "ride" suddenly ended and I ran out of conveyor belt! My feet hit that metal bar and the rest of me went flying and I landed sprawled out on the floor with my feet and arms flailing and Dill just standing there looking at me stunned, like he really didn't see what just happened. I am not sure if it scared me, hurt me, or just embarrassed me but needless to say I didn't make eye contact with anyone after that.

We finally were on our way to Athens. Our flight out of Germany was wild! That pilot was zipping around in that huge airbus like it was a Volkswagen. He would rush forward and then slam on the brakes on the runway, haha. When he took off, it was so fast that all the passengers were plastered against the seats! It was like being on an amusement ride. We went up, down, turned, dipped. The people around us were laughing and shouting, "wheeee!"

It was early morning as we flew over the Alps and they were poking through the clouds they were so tall! They were completely covered in thick snow. It was like what you would imagine heaven to be like. We then flew over the boot of Italy and we were low enough that we could see the rolling hills and vineyards. The water between Italy and Greece was so blue that it nearly took my breath away.

When we landed, our luggage was the first to come off the pick-up and we walked to the main part of the airport and right into my friend! Our Greek adventure had finally begun.

A few days later

I am sorry for not recording everything but my friend had a full agenda for us! Her kids are precious and her home was beautiful. She and her husband surprised me and Dill by giving us their bedroom, which was all cream colored, with netting over the bed and a balcony with a mountain view on one side and the sea on the other. We shopped in the markets, went to eat authentic Greek food, visited downtown Athens, somehow by the grace of God found one particular restaurant we were looking for (another book there), went swimming in the Aegean sea, and of course visited the ruins. The ruins were spectacular and I couldn't possibly find the words to describe the way it felt walking on such ancient ground. One day we rented a tiny European car and toured the island of Andros with the windows down and listened to Greek music on the radio. We spent the night at my friends' family's hotel overlooking the sea and watched fisherman catch squid from our balcony.

The highlight for me was the trip we made to Tinos. When you leave the ferry, there is a carpeted path up the hill, along the side of the street where pilgrims would crawl in reverence on their hands and knees until they reached the cathedral at the top of the hill. I felt so moved when we entered the courtyard that even though our time was limited, I wanted to go in and have the priest bless me. I had to wait through two baptisms to be noticed and then I was told that I would have to go to the end of a tremendously long line. I carried with me a note about my medical problems that had been translated and rewritten for me into Greek.

I showed the priest the letter, he read it, and led me out of the building, around a corner, and to a narrow passageway that ended in a small, dark altar. I knelt down and waited and soon another priest, this one with different colored garments came and told me that he couldn't bless me because he was only allowed to bless those who were Orthodox. I sank down and just cried. It was time to leave to board the ferry back to Athens and I felt defeated and rejected. It was at that moment that someone gently touched my shoulder and I heard a soft, compassionate voice say, "God loves everyone." I looked up into the face of an elder priest, more lavishly clothed than any. He read my note and placed it back into my hand. Then he covered my head with his robes and chanted. He anointed my head with oil and told me that God would always be with me. I think I floated away thanking God for such a surreal experience.

There are too many details about our trip to go into here, but it was the honeymoon of a lifetime. The flights back were good and we arrived in the US just when the fall leaves were turning. One night when we were in Greece, we took a taxi and the driver was trying to tell us something but there was a huge language barrier. He was doing something with his hands and saying "America, Boom, Boom, Boom." We went through our repertoire of Greek words and couldn't figure out what he could possibly be talking about until later. We came home to news about the DC sniper killings and realized that's what the driver was trying to tell us. So instead of traveling the beltway, we drove back to SC through the mountains. We actually saw black bears in the mountains and it was gorgeous with all the trees changing color.

October 25

When I was working on this book I asked my sister Bobbi to read it first and give me input. She said that her only criticism was that she felt like I breezed over my life after I found out I was terminal. She reminded me of all the ups and downs I had emotionally and physically. I didn't write in my journal for a very long time because either I was too preoccupied with living my life to it's fullest, I was writing the first part of this book, or I was too sick to do anything. There was a while that I didn't even stand up except to go to the bathroom because my equilibrium was gone. At that time, I could not write nor type. I lost my ability to record my thoughts for a long time. It is very difficult to remember a year's worth of time. This time I didn't have much solitary time like I did before when I was journaling every week sometimes more than once a day. Dill took Family Medical Leave for several months and was home with me all the time. I am so grateful for this time that we spent together.

Dr. Steinberg suggested that I contact Hospice in order to set up home care. Although I didn't feel like I needed that, I did it anyway. I became friends with my nurse who used to bake my dog bone shaped biscuits nearly every week! She was so sweet. She couldn't believe how healthy I looked and how good my attitude was and she suggested that maybe I get another opinion. So I did. But it wasn't until I felt I had no choice that I did. My headaches suddenly began to get worse and I could tell my health was failing. I had stopped juicing because Dill went back to work and I couldn't stand in the kitchen to do it because my back hurt so badly from all the weight gain caused by the steroids I was taking.

I went to see a team of doctors at the nearest medical university 100 miles away and they offered me options that I didn't realize existed for me. During the time between my revealing oncologist's visit and finding a new medical team, I can honestly say that I did really good during the times that my life had some semblance of meaning and I ate right, juiced, took my supplements, and prayed. Basically, I could tell the difference in the times that I had a lackadaisical attitude and the times when I really focused on getting well. I had lots of ups and downs. There was a while when I felt sorry for myself. It had been so long since my diagnosis that I began to think people around me either took me for granted or got tired of waiting for me to die.

October 29

I had an appointment with Dr. Monroe today at the radiation center. A really sweet volunteer picked me up and drove me. She worked for a company that was hired by the American Cancer Society to provide transportation to those who cannot drive. We got along and talked a lot. I had not thought about my volunteering for a long time until I saw how happy it made her. When we got to Dr. Monroe's office, a lot of people were really surprised to see me walking. He is so nice. This is the first time in a while I have not been in a wheelchair so he asked if he could walk me out. He put his arm around me and said, " I don't really need to see you again but if you come back we can just chat." I thought that was cute. So I made an appointment for January 2004! When they gave me the appointment card, I just stared at the date and shook my head in awe. I really didn't think I'd be around this long. God is good.

November 17

My son just turned 11 yrs. old. I can't believe it. It seems like yesterday that I was pregnant with him. How time flies. The kids had a fun weekend with sleepovers and spending time playing with their friends. My weekend wasn't so good. I try and do as much as I can and sometimes I overdo it. Dill is really doing a lot…a lot of things he is not used to doing and he is doing a pretty good job. Any marriage is hard, but when you add a major illness it compounds things. I have my own way of doing things and so does Dill and they're not always the same. But I try and respect our differences. After all, he has been my knight in shining armor and the one person in my life that knows everything I've been through and has helped me in the worst of it all.

I want to do so many things but I have to depend on others for everything. It is so frustrating for me. I am not in denial but I've been alive so much longer than the doctors told me I would that there have been times that I really didn't think about the cancer much. Because the tumors were not growing, the doctors were baffled. They did brain surgery on me last November to remove the largest of the tumors and examine it in pathology. I did exceptionally well in surgery. I was more nervous getting prepped than in my previous surgeries because this one was so serious. The preparations were pretty much the same as in all the other ones. My surgeon did not shave my head and just did surgery around the hair and then didn't bandage it. I thought this was odd but I was glad I didn't have to have that section of my hair shaved off! The nurses told me that my doctor had the lowest rate of post surgery infection than anyone in the neurology dept. and they believe this has something to do with it.

They wheeled me into surgery and I remember absolutely nothing about it before I woke up in recovery. I was hungry! They brought me spaghetti in the recovery room… I couldn't believe it, haha. When I got into a room I had a catheter and they told me they weren't sure how long I would be there. It would depend on how well I handled coming back after surgery. I hounded them constantly to bring me juice and water and by that evening they were talking about maybe the possibility of me only having to stay a little while because my body was eliminating every ounce I put in it and I wasn't feeling much pain.

I had a wonderful male nurse. I remember when the guy from the recovery room introduced me to him he said, "This remarkable young lady looked just like this when she came out of surgery. She is a really good patient". My nurse spent a lot of time in my room chatting with Dill and me.

Bobbi and her husband were there too and we were all really surprised when my nurse came in the next morning and asked me if I wanted to get out of there! I was like, "yeah!" He made some sort of arrangements for me. He said he pulled a few strings. I was home within 24 hours of having brain surgery!

It was indeed breast cancer but they still don't understand why I am alive. I went home after surgery even before my doctor made his rounds so I didn't even see him until I went back for my follow-up. Dill and I walked into the room and he said, "Now which one of you had brain surgery two weeks ago?" They made me feel really good about how well I was doing. He asked me how I felt and I jokingly said, "I feel like some drilled through my head with a power drill." He started laughing and said, "That's exactly what I did." When I heard this, I almost passed out. I was only kidding and didn't realize he cut through my skull until then! For some reason, I thought he said he was going to go underneath from my neck. Anyway, that's when I started having discomfort, only when I realized the extent of the procedure! That just goes to show you that your mental attitude can have a huge effect on how you feel. Had I known that I had just had my skull drilled open, there is no way I would have had the motivation to come home from the hospital so soon! Like they say, sometimes ignorance is bliss.

They kept me on the steroids and they caused me to continuously gain weight. During my recovery and over the next couple of months it got so bad that I could hardly swallow there was so much fat around my neck. I couldn't sleep in the bed anymore because my back hurt so badly that I couldn't lie flat. We had to buy a recliner for me to sleep in. I was up to 257 lbs. from the 165 I was when all this started. For a while I was in a wheelchair. I wanted to get off the steroids and get back on my program so I could start losing weight in order to feel better again. Things would get worse before they got better though.

I had my brain surgery around Thanksgiving and it was probably in late December or January that I felt like I was finally over the surgery. I took it easy and let people wait on me. I had stopped juicing and doing my program when I had surgery. I hadn't gotten back on it and I felt guilty about it, but I just wanted to do as little as possible. I was being really irresponsible in neglecting my body. I was relying strictly on my medical team and wasn't doing anything for myself. I looked into the latest treatments options for patients with brain mets. My mother in law had known someone who had gone to a cancer center in NY and been treated using stereo tactic radiation for the same condition as me. I ordered materials from the hospital to make the decision. This procedure was radiation but directed in a pencil thin line to the exact location of the mass. I finally decided I wanted to do it. I hated radiation but this was supposed to be different.

Looking back I think I was depressed during this time. When I first was told my prognosis, it was okay. My attitude was good and I was like a firecracker, determined that nothing would stop me. Everyone marveled at how well I was doing, but lately I had become too passive. Time was taking its toll on me. I decided I wanted to go off the steroids. I was tired of being so fat. I knew they were to keep the swelling down in my brain and so I ordered some anti-inflammatory herbs off the Internet. I didn't realize that I couldn't just stop taking them but I did. cold turkey.

Dill's mom came down in February and while she was here I took a turn for the worse. I was in bed the whole time and throwing up. I was so nauseated and my head hurt so badly I could hardly move. Everyone around me thought that I was in my final days that the end had come. I could no longer write, read, or type. I couldn't turn my head to either side because it would make me too dizzy. When I was riding to go to my doctor visits, I had to close my eyes because the objects whizzing by would overload my senses. I could barely get out of the bed to go to the bathroom and had talked to my in home care nurse about bringing a bedside potty for me because I simply couldn't make it by myself anymore to the bathroom, which was about ten feet from my bed. I had become incontinent and was seriously considering buying adult diapers.

Finally Dill came to me and begged me to go back on my steroids. I gave it a lot of thought and said I would start taking them again because I didn't want to be so sick and even though I despised the way the steroids made me feel, being off of them was worse and I just couldn't do it anymore.

When I went back to taking them, I immediately began to improve. By the end of March I was feeling much better but I still had the side effects from the weight gain. By now I had huge purple stretch marks all over my body and I could barely walk. An MRI showed that the largest brain tumor had grown back and this time was larger than before. I may have waited too late to have stereo tactic radio surgery. That was frightening to me. It took a while communicating with the hospital before my insurance company finally decided that they could not pay for the treatment since it wasn't in my home state! The only option at this point was to consider what treatment I could have locally.

I asked for an appointment with the radiation oncologist and went to see him. He performed a technique called gamma knife that was similar to the treatment I had decided I wanted so I said I would do that instead. Unfortunately, by the time I had done this, the MRI revealed that the brain tumor had grown back, bigger than it was before, and too big to have this procedure done effectively. I was so disappointed. My only option now was whole head radiation, the thing I had sworn from the beginning that I would rather die than have.

So reluctantly in May I started whole head radiation. It was very brief, only ten days but it was like ten days of hell. A cast was made of my head. During my treatments, I would have to lie flat and motionless on a metal table with my head strapped down to it inside this "cage". I would squeeze my eyes shut and when they turned the beam on, I would say" burn baby burn" to myself. I could "see" the radiation as it illuminated the inside of my head with a bright, bluish-purple light. I could make out the outline of blood vessels, I think from my eyes while this was happening, and I smelled an odor similar to charcoal. Imagine how hard this became when my head began to swell from the treatments, making the mask tight, and having to be strapped with my mouth mostly covered during a time when I thought I was going to vomit any second.

Those treatments were the worst thing I had ever been through. I was so weak I couldn't stand. When I would try to get out of the wheelchair to stand on the scales or to get up on the table, it took all the strength I had. One day I toppled off the scales and nearly hit the floor but the nurse and the technician caught me before I came into contact with the ground.

One night I had to get some water to drink because I was so dehydrated and I made it to the kitchen but fell when I got there. It was the middle of the night and all I could do was yell for Dill (who sleeps like a log) and hope that he would hear me. I did wake him up but when he tried to help me get off the floor I couldn't. I just didn't have enough strength. I finally crawled on painfully swollen knees to the living room carpet and pulled myself up, with his help, on a chair. Things got so bad that I wanted to stop going to radiation. I called them one morning and said I just couldn't go because I was too sick and weak. They gave me a day off. It was on Friday and by Monday I was rested enough I was willing to try it again.

Having my head radiated caused my hair to fall out again. This makes the third time now. But I cared less about being bald than the times before because I was so glad that I had made it through the radiation. Recovering from the radiation was slow but I rested a lot, drank a lot of water, and started taking my supplements again. I began adding juice to my diet to flush out the toxins from having the treatment. I finally began to feel better but I later found out that the whole head radiation had not had an effect on the cancer.

Talk about a wasted effort....I was so sad about this. When my doctors saw the results, or rather the lack thereof, they offered to put me on chemo again. I wasn't thrilled about this idea, but it was the only thing they knew to do. They would try a tablet form of chemo called Xeloda.

The thought of having to go through all those blood tests again was really unappealing to me. It caused me to remember going through chemo the first time and how the lab techs would draw my blood by pricking my fingers because my veins were collapsed from all the chemo IV's. They would alternate fingers to avoid sticking the same one all the time and I can remember having little scabs all over the ends of my fingers.

Not long after I started back on chemo, they began to wean me off the steroids. They lowered my dosages several times in an effort to take me off slowly. I started juicing again and watching my nutrition. I began to feel better. My hair was sprouting around the edges but not on the top and Dr. Monroe said it was because that was the location of the highest concentration of radiation I received and if I wanted, he could teach me how to do a comb-over like his! I thought that was really funny.

Anyway, I was making progress. Honestly, the more I take care of myself, the better I feel. I am slowly working towards doing more in my life. I am now starting to lose weight. So far I have lost around fifty pounds. My hair finally starting growing. I dare not say I am trying to get things back to "normal" because I have learned through all of this that there is no such thing. I have started volunteering again working a crisis line for a spousal abuse organization. I have a website on the internet offering counseling online, I am enrolling in a continuing education program that I can do mostly from home, and I have organized a breast cancer support group. I take my story to whoever will listen and I have been asked to share with other groups of people. I try to make myself available for this because I don't want the experience and the knowledge I've gained to be wasted.

Only God knows what my future holds. I am returning slowly to the outside world and find that life holds a lot of fascination. I am able now to take the time to be a curious observer of my world.

<u>January 1, 2004</u>

I can hardly believe it is 2004. In 2002 my oncologist warned me not to drive myself home from my doctor's appt. with him because I could have a seizure and I thought about this today when I was driving to the grocery store. ☺ Am I afraid I will die? No. I know that I will one day but death doesn't feel like a dark cloud following me around. Death is natural. Life is temporary and I think how we die has a lot to do with how we live. I believe my death will be a peaceful transition from this earthly life to the next, whatever that is. I believe this because I have come to terms with death. I have accepted that it will happen one day and in the meantime I am trying to enjoy my life as much as possible. I am trying always to take advantage of the opportunities that come along for me to help others and experience a higher level of existence. I see having the time to be available to others as a blessing. I believe I have finally found what it is that I was born to do. To help others unselfishly, without expecting anything in return. To do this requires having enough faith in God to know that my needs will be met, no matter what they are. It doesn't matter how long I do it but that I achieved the discovery of it.

This will probably be my last entry here because I am ready to compile all this together and hopefully find a publisher. What about the cancer? Well, according to medical science the last MRI I had showed that instead of having at least 15 tumors I now only have 4 and the largest of these (the one I had brain surgery on which had grown back) has now begun dying from the inside out. It is about 85% gone. I have been told by the doctors that I will be on chemo for the rest of my life but I don't necessarily believe the medical community anymore. What do I credit this wonderful change to? I believe it is a combination of things: the traditional treatments, my alternative therapy, and lots and lots of prayer. I think I have been given a miracle. I believe that I received my reward for taking action against this disease and doing my best to try and do everything I could to have faith and fulfill my purpose in life. God made me and only he knows when my mission is complete. Besides…it's not about how long you live but what you do with the time you are given.

Staying Motivated

If you have read my journal, you have seen that the times I let myself take a break from fighting were the times that I would end up depressed and despondent. Those were the times that I would go downhill. My largest brain tumor grew back when it was removed even after I thought I had an understanding of cancer. *Understanding what is happening and trying to do everything you can to stop it are two entirely different things.* All this knowledge does you no good if it is not put into action. It is easy to slip back into your old habits and old patterns of eating and living. It is easy to tell yourself that you have worked hard and you deserve a break. Just keep in mind the times you are taking a break from helping your body fight disease, the disease-causing problems are not taking a break. Every second you are alive your body is regenerating. It is either moving towards life or towards death. Every bite you eat and everything you come into contact with can tip that balance. You can make choices that either support the body or work against it. That part is up to you.

Read this book as often as you need to and do some research on your own. Every time you feel like you have done enough, refer to one of your research tools that will encourage you to keep trying. Remember that it may have taken cancer years to develop in your body and so it may take years to reverse it. Never give up. The one thing I promised to myself and those closest to me was that I might lose the battle in the end but one thing was for sure: I would go down fighting. *And that's what I intend to do.*

Please share this book with anyone that you think may benefit from it and thank you for giving it a chance. If you would like to email me with questions or concerns please do so at bjhenson@sccoast.net. I will try to answer every email.

Vegetarian recipes

I would just like to caution you that a lot of these recipes contain dairy products and fat. I would only eat cooked food at the main dinnertime meal and make sure that it was mostly vegetarian, *after you have fasted for at least two weeks and spent a few days eating live foods to ease your body back in the swing of normal digestion.*

Apple and grape salad

2 c Apples, cubed
1 c Grapes, halved
1/2 c Celery, chopped
1/4 c Walnuts, chopped
1 t Lemon juice
1/3 c Sour cream
1/3 c Plain yogurt

In large bowl, combine apples, grapes, celery, walnuts and lemon juice. Mix yogurt and sour cream. Mix lightly into fruit mix. Refrigerate. If desired, serve on lettuce lined plates.

Artichoke pasta salad

1c tri-color Rotini pasta or whole wheat pasta
6oz marinated artichoke hearts
1 can whole baby mushrooms
1c halved cherry tomatoes
1c med pitted ripe olives
1 lemon
1T parsley
½ t dry basil
2 T Olive oil

Cook macaroni according to package; drain well, rinse with cold water and drain again. Pour into a large bowl. Add artichokes and their liquid, mushrooms, cherry tomatoes, olives, parsley and basil; toss gently. Cover and refrigerate for at least 4 hours. Before serving, season with salt and pepper to taste and cover with lemon juice and olive oil. Toss and serve.

Asparagus casserole

1 can chopped asparagus
1 can tiny green peas
1 can cream mushroom soup
2 C. grated sharp cheddar cheese
4 hard boiled, sliced eggs

Mix asparagus, peas, soup and cheese together. Place in casserole dish. Top with eggs and heat to bubbly.

Asparagus Soup

8 oz butter
1lb asparagus spears, hard bits peeled, chopped
1 onion, roughly chopped
1 leek, roughly chopped
2-3 celery stalks
8 oz plain flour
4pt vegetable stock
Seasoning

Melt the margarine in a pan. Add the vegetables and sweat them out until they are soft. Stir in the flour a little at a time to avoid lumps. Boil for an hour and then blend it and put back on the stove for a little while. Serve with croutons.

Bean Salad

1 can cut green beans
1 can yellow beans
1 can red kidney beans
1 can garbanzos
1 can of lima beans
1 med. onion cut in rings
1 small bell pepper (any color)
1/4-1/2 c. sugar
1/3 c. salad oil
2/3 c. vinegar
1 t. salt and dash of pepper
Drain cans of beans. Mix beans, onions and bell pepper, set aside. Mix together remaining ingredients and add to the salad. Chill several hours before serving.

Beans and Rice

Large can of mixed beans or red kidney beans
One large potato, cubed
5 ripe tomatoes
1 large onion
Cumin
chili
Oregano
Paprika
Soy sauce
Pepper
Olive oil

Chop onions finely and sauté in olive oil until translucent. Add cubed potatoes and spices; cook until potato is slightly browned. Add chopped tomatoes and cook for 8-10 minutes with lid on, stirring occasionally. Add beans and chili and soy sauce to taste. Serve on rice with green salad.

Beet Salad

4 beets
3 T olive oil
1 orange
1 1/2 tsp. vinegar
3/4 t. grated ginger
1/4 cup pecan halves, broken in half lengthwise

Scrub the beets, and cover loosely with tin foil. Place on a baking sheet, and drizzle with 1 T olive oil. Bake in pre-heated 425 degree oven until tender, which should take about an hour. Then cool them in the fridge, peel, and quarter them. Peel ½ the orange and cut half the orange in segments, and then cut them crosswise. Place in a bowl and add the juice from the other half of the orange. Add vinegar and ginger and whisk in 2 T. olive oil. Add the beets to the vinaigrette and orange segments. Add the zest and the pecans, using some of the pecans as a garnish. Chill for half an hour for the flavors to mingle.

Black Bean Soup

2 cans black beans
1 lemon
4 garlic cloves, chopped
2 stalks celery, chopped
1 large chopped onion
1 can chicken broth
1 T olive oil
1 t. Tabasco sauce
½ cup ketchup
1 can whole tomatoes
2-4 jalapeno rings
Salt and pepper

Sauté onion, garlic and celery in oil. Add beans and water if needed. Combine other ingredients and simmer for an hour.

The peppers make it hot so experiment with these to suit you!

Broccoli casserole

Pkg. Frozen chopped broccoli
1 can cream of mushroom soup
2 C. mild grated cheddar cheese
Crushed Ritz crackers for topping
Small onion, chopped
Salt and pepper
1 egg

Cook broccoli and drain. Add soup, cheese, onion, salt and pepper, and egg. Stir well press into casserole dish. Top with cracker crumbs and bake until brown.

Burritos

Filling:
1 cup rice (white or brown)
1 can black beans, rinsed and drained
2 cloves crushed garlic
1-2 tsp. basil
2 Tbsp. olive oil
Salt to taste

Pico De Gallo:

3 fresh plum tomatoes, diced
2 yellow onions, chopped
1 jalapeno pepper, chopped
1/4 cup minced cilantro
1 fresh lime

Start by cooking the rice. When rice is done, add beans, garlic, salt, basil, olive oil, and mix. Let spices blend in. To make Pico de Gallo, just chop veggies, and add lime juice. To serve, pour rice mixture down the center of a 12" tortilla, top with pico de gallo, and roll up.

Cabbage Soup

Whole head of cabbage
2 Cans stewed tomatoes
Sm. Onion, chopped
1 Can Kidney beans (liquid too)
2 cloves Garlic, chopped
1 T Olive oil
Salt and Pepper
½ t Nutmeg

Chop the cabbage. Set aside. Add oil to Dutch Oven. Sautee onions until transparent. Add garlic and cook slightly but don't let it get brown. Add tomatoes (If the chunks are too big for me, I just pour them in a bowl and mash them with my fingers!) Add beans and cook for 15 min. Add cabbage and sprinkle with nutmeg. Cook until the cabbage is tender. You can eliminate the olive oil and serve this as a cold soup in the summertime. Just sauté in tomato juice.

Carrot Salad

2-3 Carrots, washed (& peeled, if you prefer)
1-2 apples, to taste
Juice of 1/2 lemon
1/2 cup raisins (optional)
1 t mayonnaise

Grate carrots, coarse or fine (or maybe a bit of both for texture?) into a bowl. Core & peel apple(s). You can either grate the apple in with the carrots, or cut into small chunks, depending on preferences. Add lemon juice, nayonaise, and raisins, if using, and mix well.

Caesar Salad

2 Heads Romaine Lettuce
Grated Parmesan Cheese
Salt And Pepper -- to taste
Juice Of 1 Lemon
1/3 Cup Garlic Olive Oil
Dash Worcestershire Sauce
2 boiled Eggs
Garlic Croutons

Wash lettuce and break into 2 to 3 inch pieces. Refrigerate for several hours. Just before serving, sprinkle generously with grated Parmesan cheese, and salt and pepper. Make dressing by combining wine vinegar, lemon juice, garlic olive oil, Worcestershire sauce, and eggs. Beat until well blended. Pour over lettuce and toss to coat. Toss in croutons and serve.

Collard greens

1 T Olive oil
Whole head washed and trimmed greens
Large rutabaga, cut into cubes
½ t Nutmeg
Salt

Cut end of collards to loosen them from bunch. Put them in sink full of cold water and sprinkle generous amount of salt. This removes sand and bugs ☺ Heat Olive oil. Add rutabagas. Thoroughly wash collards, trim tough stems, and chop. Add collards and salt liberally. Cover tightly and simmer on low to avoid burning until greens are tender, about 30 minutes.

Corn Chowder

5 medium potatoes (diced)
3 cups vegetable broth (or water)
2 tsp. olive oil
1 medium onion (diced)
3 garlic cloves (minced)
2 medium carrots (diced)
2 stalks celery (diced)
1 red pepper (diced)
1 tsp. salt
2-1/2 cups frozen corn
1 cup soy milk
1 tsp. pepper

Boil potatoes in vegetable broth or water until tender, set aside without draining. In a medium pot, heat olive oil on medium-low heat and sauté rest of ingredients except for the frozen corn and soymilk for about 5 min. In blender, blend potatoes (reserve the liquid from the potatoes) and soymilk until smooth, pour into onion and vegetable mixture with frozen corn. Stir until well mixed, add the reserved potato liquid to the pot, and cook for about 3 more min. on medium to low heat. Stir frequently.

Creamy Garlic Salad Dressing

4 ounces silken tofu (1/3 of a 12-ounce block)
4 tablespoons soymilk (1/4 cup)
1 clove garlic
1-1/2 tablespoons extra virgin olive oil
2-1/4 teaspoons vinegar
1 t Dijon mustard
1 t sugar
1 t parsley flakes
1/2 teaspoon salt
1/4 teaspoon garlic powder

Whisk ingredients until creamy smooth. Refrigerate at least 20 minutes to allow dressing to thicken, and flavors to blend.

Eggplant parmesan

1 large beaten egg
1/4 cup fat-free milk
1/8 teaspoon pepper
1 cup crushed crackers
1/4 cup grated Parmesan cheese
2 tablespoons dried parsley flakes
1 medium eggplant, sliced 1/4 inch thick
1 15-ounce can tomato sauce
1/2 teaspoon dried oregano
1 clove garlic, minced
3/4 cup shredded part-skim mozzarella cheese

In a small bowl combine egg, milk, and pepper. In another bowl stir together cracker crumbs, Parmesan cheese, and dried parsley flakes. Dip eggplant slices in the milk mixture to coat, then dip both sides in the cracker mixture. Lightly coat a 2-quart rectangular baking dish with cooking spray. Arrange eggplant in dish. In a bowl stir together tomato sauce, oregano, and garlic; pour over eggplant. Bake, covered, in a 350 degree F oven for 40 minutes or until eggplant is tender. Sprinkle with mozzarella cheese. Bake, uncovered, 10 minutes more.

Garlic Scrambled Eggs

Eggs
Milk
California Garlic Blend…garlic powder with parsley
Salt and pepper
1 T. Butter

Heat the butter, blend the eggs, milk, and spices, cook them soft and fluffy and viola! I liked to serve these with fresh sliced tomatoes and wheat toast.

Ginger Carrot Cake

3/4 cup natural apple juice
1.2 cup canola oil
1 1/2 cup raisins
1/2 cup pure maple syrup
1 1/2 cups grated carrots
2 t finely grated fresh ginger root
2 c whole wheat pastry flour
1 t baking powder
1 t baking soda
1 t cinnamon
1/2 t nutmeg
1/2 t salt
1 c chopped walnuts

Preheat oven to 350F. Lightly oil an 8x8 inch cake pan or a 9-inch round pan and dust with flour, shaking out the excess. Put the apple juice, oil, 1/2 cup of the raisins, the maple syrup, and orange zest in a blender and blend until smooth. Add the carrots and ginger and pulse just to mix. In a large bowl, whisk the flour, baking powder, baking soda, cinnamon, nutmeg, and salt together. Add the apple juice mixture and combine, using as few strokes as possible. Fold in the remaining 1-cup of raisins and the walnuts. Pour the batter into prepared pan. Use a spatula to spread the batter evenly. Bake until a toothpick inserted near the center of the cake comes out clean, 35 to 45 minutes. When the cake is done, remove from oven and let cool for 10 minutes in the pan. Transfer to a wire rack.

Greek Salad (salata)

4 ripe medium tomatoes, cored, quartered and sliced into 1 inch chunks
1 European cucumber (found in produce dept.), cut lengthwise into quarters and then slice into 1 inch chunks
1/2 c alamata olives or large black olives
6 ounces feta cheese, crumbled
1/2 red onion, thinly sliced
1 T lemon juice
2 T extra virgin olive oil
1/2 t dried oregano
Salt and pepper

Place the vegetables in a salad bowl. In a small bowl whisk together the lemon juice, oil, oregano, salt and pepper. Pour the dressing over the salad and serve.

Green bean salad

1 lb green beans, trimmed, cooked, and cooled
1 t crushed red pepper flakes
2 T rice vinegar
1 t chopped garlic
1/4 c olive oil
2 T sesame oil
2 c cherry tomatoes, halved
2 T crushed toasted peanuts
Salt and pepper

In a bowl toss all ingredients together. Season to taste with salt and pepper.

Irish potatoes

6-8 peeled and sliced potatoes
1 Stick butter

4 cups Water
Salt and pepper
Onion
Garlic
1 t. freeze-dried Chives

Just heat the butter, add the garlic, onions and potatoes to cook for 2 minutes. Salt and pepper and add the water on top. Boil down until potatoes are tender and make a thick gravy.

Jambalaya

2 c sliced okra
1 1/2 c onions, finely chopped
1 1/2 c green peppers, finely chopped
1 1/2 c celery, finely chopped
2 bay leaves
1 t salt, or to taste
1/2 t thyme
1 t oregano
1/4 t cayenne
1/2 t Tabasco
1 t garlic powder
1 c fresh chopped tomatoes
2 c converted instant brown rice
3 c vegetable stock
1/4 c chopped scallions
2 T parsley

Sauté onions, peppers and celery in 1T oil. Sauté until lightly browned. Add seasonings and continue cooking for 5 minutes, stirring frequently. Add tomato and rice. Mix well. Cook 5 more minutes. Add stock and bring to a boil. Reduce heat, cover pot, and simmer 20 minutes. Add scallions, okra and parsley. Cook 5 minutes more.

Kale and Roots

1 bunch green or purple kale
1 medium parsnip, chopped into bite-size pieces.
1 medium turnip, chopped into bite-sized pieces.
2 medium red potatoes, chopped into bite-sized pieces.
1 small yellow onion, diced.
3 cloves garlic, diced
Olive oil
Balsamic vinegar
Dash of pepper
Water

Clean kale and shop into bite sized pieces. In a large pot add a small amount of water (1/4 - 1/2 inch deep is fine). Bring water to a boil. If you have a steamer place it into the pot at this time. Put the kale, parsnip, turnip and potato into the pot. Then turn down the heat to low boil and cover the pot. In a small skillet, heat 1 - 2 tsp olive oil. Add the onion and garlic and sauté until soft. Remove the onion and garlic from the heat when done cooking. In the meantime, keep an eye on the kale and root vegetables. When the kale is thoroughly cooked and the root vegetables are soft but not mushy turn off the heat. Put the kale and root veggies in a large serving bowl. Add the onions and garlic, a swig or two or three of the balsamic vinegar (depending on how vinegary you like things), pepper to taste and toss everything together. Serve warm. This is especially good served with crusty whole wheat bread or rice or as a side dish.

Lasagna

8 dried lasagna noodles
1 10-ounce package frozen chopped broccoli
Frozen Vegetables
1 14-1/2-ounce can diced tomatoes
1 15-ounce can no salt added tomato sauce
1 cup chopped celery

1 cup chopped onion
1 cup chopped green or red sweet pepper
1 1/2 teaspoons dried basil or oregano, crushed
2 dried bay leaves
1 clove garlic, minced
1 large beaten egg
2 cups ricotta cheese
1/4 cup grated Parmesan cheese
1 cup shredded part-skim mozzarella cheese (4 ounces)
1/8 teaspoon salt
1/4 teaspoon black pepper

Cook noodles, vegetables and broccoli separately according to their package directions; drain well. Set aside. For sauce, in a large saucepan stir together tomato sauce, undrained diced tomatoes, celery, onion, sweet pepper, basil, bay leaves, garlic, and salt. Bring to boiling; reduce heat. Simmer, uncovered, for 20 to 25 minutes or until sauce is thick, stirring occasionally. Discard bay leaves. Meanwhile, for filling, in a bowl stir together egg, ricotta cheese, Parmesan cheese, and black pepper. Stir in cooked broccoli. Spread about 1/2 cup of the sauce in a 3-quart rectangular baking dish. Top with half of the noodles, half of the filling, and half of the remaining sauce. Repeat layers, ending with the sauce. Bake, uncovered, in a 350 degree F. oven for 25 minutes; sprinkle with mozzarella. Bake about 5 minutes more or until heated through. Let stand 10 minutes before serving.

Lathera – Greek Vegetables

4-5 medium size zucchini, cut in 1/4 in. disks
3-4 medium potatoes, cut in 1/4 in. disks
1-2 medium onions, sliced in thick rings
1-2 medium tomatoes, sliced in 1/4 in. disks
6-7 cloves garlic, peeled and whole
1/2 cup olive oil (or any other oil)
1/2 cup parsley

Salt and pepper
2 T oregano

Arrange in loose layers in the baking tray. Try and keep the onion rings at the bottom of the pan, they get nice and crispy, and the tomatoes go at the top of the assembly, to let the juices drain down onto the veggies bake for about 1 hour, at medium oven the oregano should be added a few minutes before taking the tray out of the oven- burnt oregano loses its flavor, and has a bitter taste. Allow to cool before eating.

Layered Vegetable Casserole

Potatoes
Carrots
Green Peppers
Mushrooms
Celery
Onions
Crushed tomatoes (optional)
1 can tomato soup
Spices (basil, parsley, oregano, garlic)

Use as many vegetables as you need to fit the chosen casserole dish. After you wash, peel and slice veggies, layer in a casserole. Between each layer, pour some soup and sprinkle with spices. Repeat until you fill dish, leaving a little room at the top. Cover and cook in the oven at 350F for 40-50 minutes or until heated through.

Lemon Pasta With Grilled Vegetables

1 box pasta
1 zucchini
15 cherry tomatoes
2 green peppers
1 large onion

5 cloves garlic
1 lemon
1-2 tsp. lemon peel
Olive oil

Chop the zucchini, onion, and green peppers into chunks and toss them in olive oil with the cherry tomatoes. Stick all the vegetables on skewers and place over a grill until partially cooked (about 10 minutes). Chop the garlic cloves up into very small cubes and sauté in oil. Grate the peel of the lemon until you have 1-2 teaspoons of lemon rind, then juice the lemon. When the pasta is done, toss it in about 1 Tbsp. of olive oil. Then add the lemon juice, lemon rind, garlic, and grilled vegetables and toss. This can also be done using sautéed vegetables instead of grilled ones.

Lima bean and artichoke casserole (this is my favorite)

1 box frozen Ford Hook (giant) lima beans
1 can artichokes (not marinated)
1 sm. onion, chopped
½ stick butter
1 can cream of celery soup
1 c grated sharp cheddar cheese
Crushed crackers
Salt and pepper

Fully cook limas until tender. Dice artichokes. Mix limas with soup, butter, artichokes, onion, and cheese. Season with salt and pepper. Pour into a casserole dish. Top with crackers, covering completely.
Heat at 350 degrees until bubbly.

Mushroom Swiss Omelet Sandwich

Fresh mushrooms
¾ stick Butter

Small chopped onion
1 T. White wine
Baby Swiss cheese slices
Rye Bread
Eggs
Salt and pepper
Miracle Whip

Melt ¾ the butter in the pan and add mushrooms and onions. Season and add wine. Cook down until tender and dark. Set aside. Melt remaining butter in pan and beat 2 eggs per omelet. Pour egg into pan and layer with cheese and mushrooms. Cook over low heat until firm, fold over and set onto rye bread spread with miracle whip. These are scrumptious!!!

Mushrooms stroganoff

1 c Vegetable Stock
2 c Onions sliced
4 c Mushrooms
1 T Paprika, sweet
Pinch Pepper, cayenne
Pinch Paprika, hot
1 t Grated lemon zest
Salt to taste
Black pepper to taste
1/2 c Yogurt, nonfat plain, strained
2 T Fresh dill

Heat 1/2 cup of the stock in a large sauté pan and add the onions. Simmer, covered, until onions are tender,10 to 15 minutes. Add the mushrooms and simmer for 5 minutes, stirring occasionally. Stir in the paprika, cayenne, lemon zest, and the remaining stock and simmer briskly for about 10 minutes until reduced by one-third (1/3). Season to taste with salt and pepper. Remove the pan from the heat and let the mixture rest for about 5 minutes, and then swirl in the yogurt. Sprinkle with chopped dill or parsley. Serve with slices of baked polenta, steamed brown or wild rice or noodles.

Oriental Greens

1 bunch baby bok choy
1/2 t salt
2 c water
1/2 T green onion, minced
1/2 T ginger root, minced
1/2 T cooking wine
1 c broth
2 t cornstarch
1 T water
1 egg white

Cut vegetables into 4-inch lengths. Heat pan with 2 cups water and 1/2 t salt until boiling. Add greens and cook for 1 minute. Remove, drain, and arrange on serving platter. Heat wok or pan and add 3 tablespoons oil. Heat until very hot. Add the minced green onion and ginger; stir-fry until fragrant. Stir-fry gently. Add the cooking wine and the broth; bring to boiling. Mix cornstarch with 1 tablespoon water. Add to mixture and cook briefly, stirring, to thicken sauce. Beat the egg white until frothy. Add in a thin stream to mixture, stirring constantly to keep egg white from setting immediately. Add 1 T oil to make it shiny (optional). Remove from heat and pour over vegetables.

Oven Roasted Potatoes

1 Envelope dry onion soup mix
2 lb Potatoes, chunked
1/3 c olive oil

Preheat oven to 450 degrees. In large plastic bag or bowl add all ingredients, close bag and shake, or toss in bowl, until potatoes are evenly coated. Empty potatoes into shallow baking or roasting pan; discard bag, bake stirring occasionally, 40 minutes or until potatoes are tender and golden brown. Garnish, if desired with chopped fresh parsley

Pea Soup

1 bag of split peas (small bag)
2 quarts of water
1 can of vegetarian chicken broth
1 carrot
1 potato
1 stalk of celery
1 onion
Salt (to taste)
Pepper (to taste)
1-2 bay leaves
Basil

Place all ingredients in a pot and cook for 2-3 hours stirring every 30-60 minutes

Peas, Potato, and Eggplant Curry

2 Large potatoes
1 med. size eggplant
1 C. frozen peas
2 cloves garlic
1 onion
Curry powder to taste
Salt and pepper

Wash and cut potatoes in small pieces. Cut eggplant into thin slices, about 2-3 inches long. Put it in water. With 2 T's of water, blend the cloves of garlic, onion, and curry powder.

Put a cooking pot over a low heat. (add oil). Add spices. When the spices become relatively thick, add potatoes. Mix thoroughly and put the lid on the pot. Let it cook 3 min. Add sliced eggplant. Mix thoroughly. Add 1/2 C. water. Put lid on. Cook for 8 min. You may want to check the veggies to make sure the bottom does not burn. Add peas and salt. Mix all veggies and put lid back. Cook for 4 to 9 min. When the eggplants feels soft, turn off the heat, mix again.

Portabella burgers

1/3 c balsamic vinegar
1/2 T rosemary
2 rolls
2 large Portobello mushrooms
4 slices mozzarella cheese
1 tomato, sliced
4 Lettuce leaves
Salt and pepper

Sprinkle mushrooms on both sides with vinegar. Salt and pepper. Place mushrooms on grill, dark gill side down. Cook until mushrooms begin to soften. Flip mushrooms. Grill until tender, about 5 minutes longer. Place cheese on mushrooms and continue to grill until melted. Assemble burgers.

Roasted Garlic

Large garlic bulbs (As many as you need)
Olive oil, ½ T per bulb
Salt
Italian bread

Preheat oven to 350 degrees. Slice the top off of the bulbs of Garlic (About 1/4 of the way from the pointy top). Drizzle olive oil on the top. Salt per taste. Wrap the bulbs in foil. Bake in oven for 2 hours. Garlic will be slightly brown on top. Serve as spread for bread that has been toast under the broiler.

Sautéed Mushrooms

Fresh mushrooms
1 stick butter
4 cloves garlic
1 lemon
Salt and pepper

Melt butter and cook garlic until tender. Add mushrooms and squeeze on lemon and spices. Cook down until tender.

Sautéed Squash

2 Zucchini
3 Yellow neck squash
1 butternut or white squash
½ C chopped onion
Chicken broth
Salt and pepper
Butter

Cut up vegetables into wheels or cubes. Heat butter and add all vegetables. Add broth and seasonings. Cook until just tender.

Spanish Rice

6 c. pre-cooked Brown Rice
1 32 oz. can chopped tomatoes, drained
1 green bell pepper, chopped
1 red bell pepper, chopped
¼ C chopped pickled jalapenos
1 large onion, chopped
2 T. mild chili powder

Olive oil
1 tsp. minced garlic
Salt and pepper

Heat large skillet and add olive oil to cover bottom of pan. Sauté onion, peppers and garlic until translucent. Add chili powder and sauté for a few minutes until heated through. Add tomatoes, jalapenos, rice and salt and pepper. Mix together until heated through.

Spinach Enchiladas

1 onion chopped
2 cloves garlic minced
3 tablespoons safflower oil
¼ C jalapeno, chopped
6 cups fresh spinach or 1 package frozen
8 corn tortillas
2 C salsa
2 C cheddar or Monterey Jack cheese, grated

In a skillet over medium heat, sauté onion and garlic in oil until golden. Stir in peppers, cook 3 minutes. Rinse spinach in water, transfer to skillet. Stir and cover, cook until wilted. Meanwhile, soften tortillas in oven, wrapped in a moist towel or foil. Place ¼ cup filling in center of each tortilla. Roll up and place seam side down in oiled ovenproof dish. Smother with salsa and cheese. Bake at 350° F until heated and bubbly.

Spinach Salad

Fresh spinach (I usually buy the bags of pre-washed because they have no sand but I wash them again anyway)

2 eggs
1 sm. Red onion, sliced in rings

½ c grated Swiss cheese
1 sm can Mandarin oranges
½ C walnut halves
Poppy seed dressing

Boil and slice the eggs. Drain the oranges. Tear the spinach into bite size pieces. Arrange on plate. Place onion slices next, then oranges, then walnuts. Drizzle with dressing and top with cheese.

Sprout sandwiches

Pita bread
Yogurt
Alfalfa sprouts
Tomatoes
Red onion
Avocado
Soy cheese

Spread yogurt inside pita pocket. Add cheese, sliced avocado, tomatoes, a few slivers of red onion and top with sprouts. The more sprouts, the better! Even my kids love these.

Squash Casserole

Pkg. Frozen chopped yellow squash
1 can cream of chicken soup
2 C. sharp grated cheddar
Pepperidge farm herbal stuffing mix
Small onion, chopped
Salt and pepper
1 C. sour cream
Stick butter

Cook squash and drain. Add soup, cheese, onion, salt and pepper, and sour cream. Blend well. Place in casserole dish and top with stuffing mix. Dot with butter and brown.

Strawberry Dump Cake

Prebaked Angel Food cake, torn into pieces
1 quart fresh strawberries, washed, trimmed and sliced
1 cup sugar
Whipped Topping

Combine wet strawberries and sugar and let set for an hour until the sugar thickens into a glaze. Place cake pieces in a bowl. Spoon glaze over cake pieces and top with Topping.

Sweet Potato Soufflé

6 baked sweet potatoes, peeled
1 T. lemon juice
1 c. brown sugar
2 cans sweetened condensed milk
1 t. cinnamon
1 t. nutmeg
1 t. vanilla extract
1 stick butter, softened

Mix well in bowl and spread into greased casserole. Cover top with layer of marshmallows and bake until brown.

Szechuan stir-fry

1 lb Tofu, cubed
½ lb Snow peas
1/3 C Teriyaki sauce
3 T Szechuan spicy stir fry sauce
2 t Cornstarch
1 Onion, chopped

3 C Chopped bok choy
2 T Cooking oil
1 C Broccoli florets
1 Red bell pepper
6 oz mushrooms
14 oz can baby corn

Combine teriyaki, stir-fry sauce and cornstarch; set aside. Cut bell pepper in strips. Cut snow peas and baby corn in half. In wok stir fry onion & bok choy in 1 T. oil for 2 minutes. Add broccoli & bell pepper; stir-fry 2 minutes. Remove from oil. Stir-fry cubed tofu in 1 T. oil for 2 minutes; add more oil if necessary. Stir sauce mixture and add to tofu; cook until bubbly. Add all vegetables; heat through. Serve over hot rice.

Tzaziki

1 European cucumber, grated
¼ c onion, grated
1 clove garlic, crushed
1 C plain yogurt
½ T lemon juice
salt and pepper
2 t basil or dill

Stir all ingredients together and chill for an hour. Serve with fresh veggies or melba toast.

Veggie Burger Patties

1 Celery stalk
1 Small onion
1 Scallion
1 Garlic clove
1 C brown rice, cooked
1 Can chick peas, drained

½ C Instant uncooked oatmeal
1/8 t Salt
1 t Paprika
½ t Dried basil
2 T Soy sauce
¼ t Ground black pepper
Olive oil as needed

Finely chop celery, onion, scallion and garlic. Set aside. In a large mixing bowl, combine the barley, chick peas, oatmeal, salt, paprika, basil, soy sauce and pepper. Mix them thoroughly with a wooden spoon or with your hands. Add the chopped celery, onion, scallion and garlic to the barley mixture and mix again. Shape into six burgers. Heat olive oil in a nonstick skillet. Add burgers and brown 5-7 minutes on each side. Or bake the patties at 350'F on a lightly oiled cookie sheet for 25 minutes. Serve on a hamburger bun with sprouts and tomato slices or ketchup.

Vegetable Pasta

1 tablespoon cooking oil
1 clove garlic, minced
2 small zucchini, sliced 1/4 inch thick (2 cups)
1 small yellow summer squash, sliced 1/4 inch thick (1 cup)
5 ounces fresh mushrooms, sliced (2 cups)
3 green onions, sliced (1/3 cup)
1/2 teaspoon dried oregano, crushed
1 large tomato, diced (1-1/2 cups)
1/8 teaspoon pepper
8 ounces corkscrew macaroni, cooked and drained
1/4 cup finely shredded Romano or Parmesan cheese
1 cup shredded provolone or mozzarella cheese (4 ounces)

Pour cooking oil into a wok or large skillet. (Add more oil as necessary during cooking.) Preheat over medium-high heat. Stir-fry garlic in hot oil for 15 seconds. Add zucchini and summer squash; stir-fry for 3 minutes. Add mushrooms and green onions; stir-fry about 1 minute more or until vegetables are crisp-tender. Add tomato, oregano, and 1/8 teaspoon pepper; stir-fry for 2 minutes more. Remove from heat. Transfer hot cooked corkscrew macaroni and Romano or Parmesan cheese to the vegetable mixture. Toss to combine. Serve immediately. Sprinkle with provolone or mozzarella cheese and freshly ground pepper.

Zucchini tomato bread

3 eggs
1 c brown sugar
1 c applesauce
3 med. Zucchini, shredded
1 chopped tomato
1 c olive oil
2 t vanilla
3 c wheat flour
½ c chopped raw sunflower seeds
1 t salt
1 t soda
1 t powder
2 t cinnamon
½ t nutmeg
¼ t cloves

Preheat oven to 325. Beat eggs, sugar, oil, and vanilla. Add remaining ingredients. Beat by hand until thoroughly mixed. Bake 50-60 min.

Write down the name of one recipe that you will try this week.

Glossary

Acidosis—a condition characterized by excessive acid in the body fluids.

Biopsy—the procedure for removing a sample of tissue in order to test it for cancer cells.

Bone marrow—soft tissue inside bones that manufactures blood cells.

Brain Stem—the part of the brain that is connected to the spinal chord.

Cancer—a term for many diseases that causes cells to grow out of control.

Cerebellum—part of the brain located in the back of the head between the cerebrum and the brain stem.

Cerebrum—the biggest part of the brain, which is divided into two hemispheres.

Chelation—the process of pulling metallic substances out of the body.

Chemotherapy—treatment with chemical agents (drugs) to fight cancer. This can be intravenous or oral.

CAT scan—an x-ray using a computer to produce pictures of the inside of the body.

Cyst—a closed sac or capsule, usually filled with fluid or material that is not solid.

Edema—swelling caused by a buildup of body fluid.

Immune system—the group of organs and cells that defend the body against infection or disease.

Lumpectomy—the surgical removal of a lump or mass.

Malignant—cancerous.

Mastectomy—the surgical removal of the breast.

Metastasis—the spread of cancer from one part of the body to another.

MRI—a test using magnetic imaging linked to a computer to produce images of the inside of the body.

Neurosurgeon—a doctor who specializes in performing surgery on the brain.

Oncologist—a cancer specialist.

Pathology—the study of identifying diseases.

Prognosis—the probable outcome of a disease.

Radiation—a medical procedure whereby a radioactive substance or very strong light is used to kill cancer cells.

Recur—to come back again.

Steroids—drugs used to relieve inflammation.

Tumor—an abnormal mass of tissue.

Vermafuge—substance that is designed to expel parasites out of the body.

If there are terms which you do not know the meaning of, or topics that you are confused about, write them down and do research to find the answers. Talk to your doctor, surf the Internet, visit the library, or bookstore.

Knowledge is power!

Made in United States
North Haven, CT
05 November 2026

21775928R00161